The
Resolution
Diet

The Resolution Diet

David Heber, MD, PhD

AVERY PUBLISHING GROUP

Garden City Park • New York

The information, advice, and procedures contained in this book are based upon the research and the personal and professional experiences of the author. They are not intended as a substitute for consulting with your physician or other health care provider. The author and publisher urge all readers to be aware of their health status and to consult health care professionals before beginning any health or fitness program, including changes in dietary habits and physical activity.

Cover designer: Doug Brooks
In-house editor: Lisa James
Typesetter: Gary A. Rosenberg
Printer: Paragon Press, Honesdale, PA

Avery Publishing Group
120 Old Broadway
Garden City Park, NY 11040
1–800–548–5757
www.averypublishing.com

Publisher's Cataloging-in-Publication

Heber, David.
    The resolution diet : keeping the promise of
permanent weight loss / David Heber — 1st ed.
        p. cm.
        Includes bibliographical references and index.
        ISBN: 0-89529-872-4

    1. Reducing diets. 2. Weight loss. I. Title.

RM222.2.H43 1999   613.2′5
                                                    QBI98-1564

Contents

To my family and relatives,
my patients, and my friends
for all their support,
and to all those who would like to
lose weight safely and effectively
once and for all.

Acknowledgments

I would first like to thank my patients, who taught me on a weekly basis in clinic what was important to them, what worked for them, and how I should mold the nutrition and behavior-science messages that I employed to help them. I also want to thank all of those who worked with me at UCLA, including Dr. Roslyn Alfin-Slater, Dr. Judith Ashley, Dr. Dilprit Bagga, Dr. Shlalender Bhasin, Dr. Jo Anne Brasel, Dr. Lauri O. Byerley, Dr. Karen Duvall, Dr. Vay Liang W. Go, Dr. Lindsey Henson, Dr. Michael Hirt, Dr. Zhaoping Li, Dr. Edward Livingston, Dr. Morton H. Maxwell, Dr. Susan Stangl, Dr. Marion Swendseid, Dr. Ronald Swerdloff, Dr. John Tayek, Dr. Herbert Weiner, Dr. Joel Yager, Dr. Ian Yip, and Dr. Marjorie Yong— along with my medical students, interns, and residents; nurses and staff; dietitians; exercise physiologists; and psychologists— who struggled with me to establish this field within traditional medicine using a scientific approach. This effort culminated in the establishment of the UCLA Center for Human Nutrition.

I especially want to thank Susan Bowerman, M.S., R.D., Executive Assistant to the Director of the Center for Human Nutrition, and Pamela Saltsman, M.P.H., R.D., Chief Research and Clinical Dietitian at the center, for reviewing the manuscript intensively with me for nutrition-education content and meaning, both explicitly and between the lines.

A special thanks goes to my loving wife, Anita, and my children, Marc and Adrianna, who put up with my spending hours in front of the computer working on this book when I should have been spending time with them.

Finally, I would like to thank my publisher, Mr. Rudy Shur, and my editor, Ms. Lisa James, for their hard work and help in editing this manuscript.

David Heber, M.D., Ph.D.
Los Angeles, California

Preface

Many of us are born with the tendency to store any extra calories we eat as body fat. This trait has been bred into us. While humans have been on this planet for 50,000 years, during most of that time food has been scarce. In response to that scarcity, our bodies have been programmed to store calories against possible future starvation. Agriculture only developed 10,000 years ago, and modern food production has been in place for less than 100 years. In the last fifty years of relative prosperity in industrial nations, we have produced a huge surplus of food while also creating a high-stress, inactive lifestyle. Our bodies haven't had time to adjust. This has set the stage for an epidemic of obesity.

Therefore, it is no wonder that more of us are overweight than ever before. When we eat the foods all around us that taste good, such as fast foods and high-fat, high-sweet desserts, without thinking of the long-term effects they have on our bodies, we end up gaining weight. If you have gotten caught up in this epidemic and find that you have to struggle to control your weight, this book is for you.

The good news is that research on nutrition and behavior has proven that permanent changes in eating habits can work, *if* you approach this problem in the right way. Simplistic diets based on "easy" solutions may organize your eating habits for a few days or weeks, but these approaches don't work for long. In this book, I have combined the best of nutrition science and behavior science into a simple approach that works. This approach will make it possible for you to lose weight and keep it off, once and for all. You will start by deciding why you want to lose weight, and how much you should expect to lose. After personalizing your weight-loss plan, you will learn what foods and what thoughts are keeping you from losing weight, and how you can change. You will learn how to control your eating with meal replacements and portion-controlled foods, and you will learn key strategies to keep you on your plan in restaurants and other high-risk places. You will also learn the right kinds of exercise that will allow you to burn off fat every day, and the right kinds of thoughts to prevent you from falling back into your old eating habits.

While all this new information about nutrition is interesting, you have to apply the things you have learned in your everyday life to make them work. From day one, you will be applying your new knowledge so that you can lose weight. As in other areas of life, there are "different strokes for different folks." You will learn how to combine the various approaches I provide you to make this plan your own. Your Resolution Diet will contain only those elements that apply to you personally, and you will work your way through the book with questionnaires, called profiles, that highlight what applies to you.

I have personal, professional, and public-service reasons for writing this book. You see, I was an overweight kid. I wore a portly suit at age thirteen and had close friends, both male and female, who suffered the loss of self-esteem that comes from being thought of as unattractive or undesirably overweight. Overweight people are often thought of as lazy or as having no self-control, and many people look at you differently if you are overweight. As a kid, I would eat a big plate of French fries and a hamburger for dinner almost every night, and my body stored the fat away.

I did something about my weight a long time ago. In my senior year at UCLA in 1969, I lost twenty-five pounds by eating what was then considered a diet—cottage cheese and canned peaches, hamburger patties with no bun, and a low-fiber puffy cereal that was mostly air. I also ran around the track every day. I never regained those twenty-five pounds.

Over the years, I have learned much more about nutrition, and over the last twenty-three years I have treated thousands of patients at the UCLA Medical Center. I have treated patients at every economic level, of many different racial and ethnic backgrounds, and from every walk of life, including Hollywood celebrities, politicians, lawyers, businessmen, and housewives. If they can lose weight, so can you.

While I remain confident about my ability to help people one on one, I want to do more. By writing this book, I believe I can help people like you. If you are ready to change, and need the inspiration to do so, this book is for you. If you don't know what to do with all the new magic pills, potions, and exercise equipment, then this book is for you. Finally, if you are severely overweight and you are going to be working with your doctor, you can use this book as a source of information for both of you. I teach physicians all the time, and your doctor will find the information here credible and up to date. My goal in writing this book is to make you an expert on yourself.

We all have bodies of different shapes and sizes, and with different amounts of body fat. What is your personal story? How can you easily and safely control your body fat? You have to visualize where you are going. So let's get started on developing a vision—a vision of a slimmer, healthier you.

Introduction

If you feel as though you have spent a lifetime dieting and not losing weight, take heart. The Resolution Diet is about the good news that you can lose weight, and keep it off, permanently. This book will provide you with the information you need to tailor a diet, exercise, and stress-reduction plan to the life you live.

I know it seems like there's a new diet every week. But most diets don't work for long because they don't give you all the tools you need to lose weight. The information in this book is based on the latest scientific understanding of the fundamental nature of weight gain and loss. Most human disorders, including being overweight, have many different causes, and this book will help you understand the many factors in your life that contribute to the additional pounds you are carrying around. This includes the most important factor of all—the changing nature of food in this country as a source of profit, rather than a source of nourishment. Food marketing can influence you so that you lose your common sense about eating. This book will help you regain that sense.

The Resolution Diet will teach you to take responsibility for your new lifestyle by recognizing that you may not be perfect

In *The Resolution Diet*, I will first help you get ready to make your weight-loss promise to yourself. I will show you why it is more important to learn about the links among food, behavior, and biology than it is to simply follow some "eat this, don't eat that" type of diet. I will help you educate your palate, so you understand why you eat the way you do, and why exercise is so important. Finally, I will teach you ways to keep your promise so that your personal diet resolution can become a permanent way of life. All along, the profiles will help you put what you learn into action. And to help you learn for a lifetime, I have a website address that serves as an online support group and lets you stay abreast of the latest nutrition research.

So let's deal with being overweight as a problem that is keeping you from being the healthiest person you can be. The good news is that you can do some simple things to help yourself conquer this problem and live a thinner, healthier life.

Chapter 1

A Step-By-Step Weight-Loss Resolution

When it comes to nutrition, you have probably heard a lot of different and sometimes conflicting advice: "just count carbs," "just count fat grams," "calories count," "calories don't count," "eat more, weigh less," "eat more protein," "balance your protein, carbohydrates, and fats," "never eat carbohydrates with protein," "all you need to do is exercise," "all you have to do is think yourself thin," "don't deprive yourself," "eat what tastes good," "fat is beautiful," and finally "diets don't work." It's enough to send you to the drive-through!

Over the past twenty years, I have worked with thousands of patients to help them lose weight and keep it off. During this time, I have combined my knowledge of nutrition science with what these people have told me worked for them. The program I am about to offer you is one you will mold to fit your own lifestyle and individual needs.

WHY ARE WE GETTING FATTER?

For the most part, there are four basic reasons why we are getting fatter as a society—the hidden fat and calories in our diet, our basic genetic blueprint, increased stress, and lack of physical activity.

You may have been eating high-fat, high-calorie foods— foods that someone else has designed to deliver good taste at the lowest possible price—without thinking through the long-term effects on your body. Your friends and neighbors have also voted for these foods with their palates, since taste determines how well foods sell. At the same time, we have lost our common-sense approach to eating, which means just eating when we are hungry. Instead, our eating behaviors reflect the advertising message that the more we eat, the more fun, friendship, and love we will have. In fact, there are many situations where we finish off bowls of potato chips, corn chips, or other snack foods without even focusing on what we are eating. In other words, we are eating unconsciously not because we are hungry, but because we are in a situation that calls for munching on something. We eat when we are happy, sad, lonely, stressed, or relaxed, or in a variety of social situations. I will do my best to point out the strategies that will work for you in these situations.

Our genetic blueprint is a wonderful one that has permitted humankind to survive starvation in many different environments. This means it has a built-in ability to conserve fat and calories, which were scarce in the environment our ancestors lived in. This genetic tendency varies from one person to another. We all know people who can seemingly eat whatever they want and not gain weight. Others look at a hot fudge sundae cross-eyed and gain four pounds! Genes confer the capability to gain weight, but your diet and lifestyle determine whether and to what extent that potential is realized.

So why else has there been a 33 percent increase in the number of overweight individuals in our country in the last decade? Stress is another factor. As a society, we have worked longer hours in the last decade, and we have had less time to take care of our personal needs. The fax machines, computers, portable phones, airline travel, and Internet, which were supposed to make our lives easier, have had the exact opposite effect. For example, an executive in the 1960s might have spent the morning making two long phone calls and dictating a letter or two before breaking for lunch. Today, executives work up to eighty hours per week, including weekends and nights. In the 1960s, a contract would be sent in the mail, and business moved on a time scale of days to weeks. Today, the contract goes out immediately and the deal is made before the end of the business day. And life is no less stressful in the mailroom or on the shop floor than it is in the boardroom. On the home front, kids used to stay after school to participate in sports. Mothers were often home, and had the afternoon to cook a big dinner for the whole family. Today, many schools no longer provide sports activities in the afternoon, and there are many more single moms juggling work and home life. So women are left to drive kids to dance, soccer, football, and baseball, all while shopping for dinner and holding a part- or full-time job. No wonder you're under stress!

When a night off finally arrives, you go out for a nice dinner, where you can completely lose control of your portions. You can easily have enough calories in one sitting at a restaurant to make up for two or three days of careful eating.

How about some exercise? If this doesn't sound appealing to you, you are not alone. About 25 percent of the population does not exercise at all. It may seem to be too much for you to drive to a gym, change, shower, change again, and drive home three times a week. Fitting exercise into your busy schedule—when we all depend more on elevators, escalators, and cars to get around—results in many fewer calories being burned each day. If you don't burn energy through exercise, you gain weight even with constant food intake.

The first thing you must recognize is that these four factors are very powerful forces that can subconsciously affect your ability to achieve and maintain a healthy body weight. You are not alone. In the United States, up to half of all women over age forty-five and a fifth of all men are dieting at any given time. I will show you how to establish a weight-loss goal, how to reach that goal, and how to maintain a healthy body weight.

MAKING YOUR PERSONAL PROMISE

We all make resolutions at one time or another. While resolutions have a mixed reputation—we all know about the New Year's resolution that is forgotten by January 3—lots of people keep resolutions successfully. Who are these people? They are the successful and effective people who periodically evaluate where they are and where they want to be. They view their resolutions as promises to themselves that must be kept. You can be one of these people if you define the day of your resolution as the beginning of the rest of your life.

We know that resolutions can work very well for people who successfully stop smoking. Those smokers who stop "cold turkey" on their own are the ones who most often are able to stop smoking for good. A nutrition resolution is more complex, because you cannot stop eating altogether. You need a method to make and keep your resolution. I will help you succeed by teaching you the secrets of successfully losing weight for good, secrets based on the latest scientific advances. I will also teach you how to make your resolution, which is really a promise to yourself that you intend to keep. In fact, succeeding at the process of making and keeping weight-loss promises will help you in other parts of your life. Let's take a look at my seven-step weight-loss resolution plan.

STEP 1: GETTING READY TO MAKE THE PROMISE

You have to be motivated to change before you make your resolution. Patients who receive gift consultations to the UCLA Center for Human Nutrition, where I work, don't change their lifestyles very much because they are not ready to change. Those who come in on their own have a higher rate of success. You need to decide which promises are the most important for you based on your personal profile, which includes your physiology, psychology, and lifestyle factors.

It is easy for so-called experts to say you should eat less and exercise more, but how? The answer to this question depends on you. How much muscle and fat do you have? Where is your fat located? Is your metabolism slow or fast? It is important to answer these questions, so you can gear your efforts towards the right things. For example, I see women who always want to lose more weight, no matter how thin they are, and who wind up losing muscle by eating poorly. Since each pound of muscle burns 14 calories a day, these women condemn themselves to a lifetime of unsuccessful dieting. You may have this problem, or your problem may lie in another area. You won't know exactly what you have to work on without an individual physiology profile.

While physiology is important, behavior is king. You need to know why you are eating the way you are now before you can change. It is also important to know how motivated you are to change. By the end of Chapter 2, you will determine your readiness to change and will save this profile for consideration in making your resolution.

STEP 2: ELIMINATING THE FOODS AND THOUGHTS THAT ARE KEEPING YOU FROM LOSING WEIGHT

There are certain foods which can keep you from losing weight. These foods are different for each person. For one it may be cheese and pizza, for another it may be red meat. For others it is nonfat yogurt and chocolate chip cookies. I call these foods and others "trigger foods." These are the foods that you are eating to relieve stress or boredom. You are not eating these foods out of hunger, but out of craving. I will show you how to identify the foods that are giving you problems.

It is also important to know the thoughts that are motivating you to eat these trigger foods. By controlling the thoughts and the foods simultaneously, you will be stopping the inflow of excess calories every day. So I have combined nutrition and behavior messages together in the Trigger Food Strategy, which is described in Chapter 3. I have learned over the years to personalize my approach to different patients. In that chapter, you will also learn how to personalize your resolution, overcome negative thought processes, and use only those strategies that will work for you.

STEP 3: TAKING CHARGE OF YOUR FOOD HABITS WITH MEAL REPLACEMENTS AND PORTION-CONTROLLED FOODS

When I talk to patients, they tell me they often don't have much time to eat properly. They are faced with food in restaurants or in social situations, so they eat even when they are not hungry. Meal replacements and portion-controlled meals can be great tools that allow you to take charge of your eating. Once you know how many calories you are eating, the weight loss will follow.

In Chapter 4, you will learn how to use these tools to lose weight predictably while learning about your eating habits. If you are someone who skips breakfast now, you will learn to eat a healthier breakfast. If you usually eat a very high-calorie lunch or dinner and that habit is keeping you from losing weight, you soon will learn to have a satisfying low-calorie lunch or dinner. If you work late at the office, you will learn that having a meal replacement can help cut down on your hunger while increasing your energy. Then you won't overindulge later in the night. If you miss a meal, you can have a meal replacement in your car instead of having fast food on the road. These strategies and others will provide you with a predictable weight loss for as many meals as you choose to control, and in those situations where you think it will help you the most. You will learn which meal replacements and portion-controlled meals are the most useful, and how to combine them with a healthy diet.

STEP 4: EDUCATING YOUR PALATE

Do you know why we eat what we eat? Humans evolved in a world where they were surrounded by fruits and vegetables that were high in fiber, high in vitamins and minerals, but low in salt, cholesterol, and fat. We like sweet foods because we are seeking the sweet taste found in fruits and vegetables. We hold onto salt, fat, and cholesterol because these were scarce in our ancient environment. In the last hundred years or so, we have been flooded with fat, sugar, and salt by the food industry, which is trying to sell us good-tasting foods. For example, they could never sell yogurt in this country until they made it taste like ice cream. This sweet, fatty treat can become your friend when you are sad or lonely, or it can be a reward for a job well done.

In Chapter 5, I will show you how to reeducate your palate to get out of this high-calorie rut. You will return to your natural tastes by eating healthier, great-tasting foods. The amazing thing is that once you go through this process, you won't be able to eat high-fat foods without being put off. I know it's hard to believe, but I have experienced it myself and seen it in my patients. You will find out about a new way of eating called the California Cuisine Pyramid that we have developed at UCLA to encourage healthier eating by everyone. You will learn how to change your eating habits once and for all.

STEP 5: LIVING THE RESOLUTION DIET

One of the great advantages of combining nutrition and behavior messages is that they are easy to remember. You see a certain set of circumstances, and you decide to use a strategy without really thinking about it. For example, a stewardess on an airline throws nuts down on your tray. You hand them back to her and say, "Tomato juice, please." If you have to consult a book to determine that there are 90 calories in those peanuts that you don't need or want, it will be too late. Or you're home after everyone has left. If you don't have a plan for eating during the day, you're in trouble.

Or you are over at Grandma's house for Thanksgiving. Are you going to eat whatever she ladles onto your plate, including gravy on her favorite mashed potatoes made with gobs of butter? Or are you going to inform her that you have started a special diet and prefer just white meat of turkey topped with cranberry sauce, some carrots, and a little bit of rice?

In Chapter 6, you will learn how to stick to your resolution in a variety of situations, from home to the office to social gatherings in restaurants and other places. These specific tactics will allow you to put the Resolution Diet to work for you now and for the rest of your life.

STEP 6: GETTING THE EXERCISE AND STRESS-REDUCTION HABITS

Our genes have been engineered for high levels of activity. This allowed our ancestors to run a step faster than the local saber-toothed tiger and to do the physical work needed to feed themselves before the development of agriculture. Ancient humans spent three to five hours a day digging for roots and other high-fiber plant foods that contained only a few calories per bite. Through evolution our bodies have adapted to this low-calorie, high-activity way of life.

With the advent of modern agriculture, the industrial revolution, and finally high-fat fast food, we no longer have this problem. Nowadays, we can get all the calories we need for the whole day in a double-double cheeseburger by digging some quarters out of our pockets. No amount of exercise will balance the amount of extra fat you can eat, if you just eat whatever you want (unless you are built like Arnold Schwarzenegger). Nevertheless, regular exercise is crucial to weight loss. For many small women, the only way to lose weight is to exercise in addition to changing the way they eat. Exercise involves a two-step process. First, you need to fit fitness into your lifestyle, to make it a habit. Then you need to build and maintain increased muscle. I will teach you how to do this in Chapter 7.

And while exercise is a great stress reducer, I will give you other tips that will help you deal with everyday stresses so that you can control your eating habits.

STEP 7: KEEPING THE PROMISE

Humans are creatures of habit. We find habits to be comforting and reinforcing. Every marketer knows this. They offer you coupons and free deals to try their food, knowing that once you get the habit of eating their food you won't stop. There used to be a famous potato chip commercial that said, "You can't eat just one!" Once you are at this stage, you have the habit. And there's no question that it's hard to break.

The information you will receive in this book is only helpful if you use it. Practice makes perfect when it comes to eating and exercise, and fitting fitness and healthy foods into your lifestyle requires the work of creating healthy habits. You will slip along the way, but I will teach you the secrets of developing good habits. This will help you stick to your resolution when the unexpected happens—a sudden assignment at work, a crisis at home, an illness, or some other uncontrollable stress. You will learn how not to let such stresses shake your resolve.

In Chapter 8, you will learn how to avoid relapses and yo-yo dieting, to stay on an even keel emotionally, to monitor your progress (and reward yourself for a job well done), and to keep refining your resolution as you go along. This will let you keep the promises you make to yourself.

MAKING IT HAPPEN

In nutrition and weight loss, as in other areas of life, you must take responsibility for yourself. You can receive help from trainers, family, and friends, but in the last analysis nobody takes better care of you than you do. As you go through the book, you will learn how to take responsibility for the promises that you make so that your resolutions will remain a reality.

The bottom line of the Resolution Diet is to put together all the profiles you have developed on your body, behavior, and promises so that you can make and keep your own personalized resolution. You will learn to save your energy and your focus for those things that are important to you personally. I will show you how your behavior can change, even in the high-fat, high-stress world we live in today.

So let's get started right now by preparing you for your resolution in Chapter 2. Let the Resolution Diet be your guide to losing weight and keeping it off, once and for all.

Chapter 2

Getting Ready to Lose Weight

There are three components to success—knowledge, attitude, and behavior. This is true no matter what you are trying to accomplish, from learning to play golf to trying to lose weight. Weight-loss knowledge that is technically correct but that encourages wrong attitudes and behaviors is of no use to you at all.

It is important to prepare your mind as well as your body for the adventure you are about experience. Just as your muscles lose their tone if you do not exercise for a long time, your mind—to say nothing of your taste buds—has settled into a comfortable, unhealthy lifestyle that you have been taught to enjoy. You have been sold on the tastes and appearances of certain foods, and on the situations in which you enjoy those foods. (Have you ever thought about the real meaning of a "Happy Meal"?) Taste, cost, and convenience are the three principles that sell food, and my job is to motivate you to ignore the sales pitch. The good news is that once you do change, you won't want to go back to your old ways.

In this chapter, I will explain how genetics and behavior affect nutrition. We will then look at the reasons people want to lose weight, and the types of weight they want to lose. I'll explain how to change the habits that sabotage your attempts to lose weight. Most importantly, I'll help you set your own personal weight-loss goal.

NUTRITION SCIENCE, BEHAVIOR, AND GENETICS

Breakthroughs in the science of nutrition, plus a better understanding of human behavior and genetics, have provided evidence that it is possible for you to finally succeed at losing weight and keeping it off. There has been a long-standing argument between those people who think being overfat is a character weakness and those who think it is an unalterable fate determined by genetics. (You can, by the way, be overweight without being overfat. Extremely muscular people often exceed standard weight-for-height guidelines, since muscle is heavier than fat.) We now know that genes determine your potential to become overfat, and that diet and lifestyle determine whether and to what extent this happens.

Genetics and Body Fat

It has been known for a long time that genes determine the shape of your face, the size of your feet, and how tall you are. We also now know that genes determine how and where you will accumulate fat. Identical twins reared in separate homes have identical distributions of fat on their bodies. That this should happen in twins reared thousands of miles apart is remarkable. We know that, through chemical messengers called hormones, the brain and the fat cell communicate with each other. So there is a genetic component to fat accumulation.

This genetic link is tied to the way your brain controls your body fat levels. The brain controls many essential body functions, such as your temperature and breathing patterns, unconsciously. In the same way, your body fat, appetite, and physical activity level are all controlled by a center in your brain called the hypothalamus. It is like a computer center that takes in all kinds of inputs and translates them into signals that control how much of an appetite you have. Did you ever consider how remarkable it is that some people's weight stays within a few pounds over many years? If your system was out of balance by just 500 calories per day, you would gain 50 pounds per year. The hypothalamus keeps this from happening. Some people, though, have their appetite thermostat set on "high," so that they eat more before they are satisfied.

The Link Between the Appetite Control Center and the Fat Cell

We know a lot about the appetite and body fat control center. It is near the center that regulates reproduction, so girls go into puberty when they reach a critical level of body fat. It is near the thirst center, which explains why so many dieters down huge bottles of water. The chemical signals in the appetite center are similar to those that affect depression. Serotonin is a pleasure-giving chemical that is low in some people with so-called "burn-out" depression, or that caused by overwork and stress. Drugs that help this condition are those that can raise serotonin levels (such as Prozac and Zoloft). Sweets can act the same way. They will indirectly raise the levels of serotonin in the brain, explaining why some people are sweet or carbohydrate cravers.

Studies with rats show how carefully the appetite center regulates body fat. If I change the pellets the rats eat to those that contain more fat, they will eat fewer pellets and maintain a constant body weight. If I decrease the amount of fat per pellet, they will eat more pellets and still maintain a constant weight. On the other hand, if I feed the rats a diet of salami, pizza, peanut butter, and chocolate chip cookies, they will lose control of their body weight and become as big as genetically obese mice. The taste factor overwhelms the appetite center. This observation was one of the factors that motivated me to develop the Trigger Food Strategy you will read about in Chapter 3 of this book.

We are learning more about the many signals that act on the appetite thermostat. We have learned that the fat cells in our bodies produce a protein called leptin, which goes to the appetite thermostat to reduce food intake. When given to obese mice, leptin causes weight loss.

It is remarkable how the fat cells and the brain are connected. When you eat, the fat cell actually makes more leptin to signal your brain that you are full and it is time to reduce appetite. People who are overfat appear to have enough leptin coming from their fat cells, but do not appear to react to it. This causes leptin levels to be higher than they should be. We know that leptin does not act alone, but works with other proteins, such as neuropeptide Y. Recently, two hormones have been identified, called Orexin A and Orexin B, that decrease food intake. If you are getting the idea that your brain is concerned with your appetite and food intake, you are absolutely right.

The first human trials of leptin, given as an injection, have shown that humans can lose sixteen pounds in six months, but much more work will need to be done before this approach is ready for general use. Companies are also working on other proteins that may be involved in appetite control. It won't surprise me if there are a number of drugs that need to be given in combination, as in the treatment of high blood pressure, to control body weight. In any case, no matter what is discovered, patients will still have to change the way they eat.

WHY DO YOU WANT TO LOSE WEIGHT?

While there are many reasons for people wanting to lose weight, they usually fall into one of these basic categories: (1) looking sexier and more attractive, (2) feeling better and stronger, or (3) getting and staying healthy. Your choice of one of these major motivators will determine both your goals and the methods you use to attain those goals.

Looking Sexier and More Attractive

You may want to lose weight to look better and be more attractive to others. There is nothing wrong with this reason.

Some doctors look down at this as "cosmetic" weight loss. But how you look—actually, how you feel about how you look—is an important aspect of life. If you feel unattractive, it affects your self-esteem, your success at work, and all of your relationships.

However, there are some pitfalls you need to avoid. Make sure it is not just someone else's problem that you are perceived as unattractive. I have seen patients who were very attractive, but who did not feel appreciated by others. Losing weight can help you feel better about yourself and permit you to wear better-fitting clothes, but it will not by itself give you self-esteem.

While you are learning and following this program, you should also be working on your emotional and spiritual side. If food is filling an emotional need, you are not going to succeed until you take some concrete steps to deal with the emotional reasons for feeling bad about yourself aside from your weight. Feeling low from time to time is pretty normal, but the accumulated damage from many insults about being overweight can lead to reduced self-esteem. I have seen patients who were successful in every area of their lives except for this one. These deep-seated emotional problems can be tackled simultaneously along with losing weight and taking on a new lifestyle.

Feeling Better and Stronger

Even though you may be taking in more calories than you should when you add up everything you eat in a day, there may be times during each day when you don't eat enough. If you skip breakfast, studies have shown that you will not be alert or able to perform, mentally or physically, in the late morning. If you skip lunch, you will not be able to perform at your best in the late afternoon, and you may feel lightheaded and edgy as the day wears on. When dinnertime comes, you may be so hungry that you not only overeat at dinner but also snack throughout the evening.

By eating healthy meals with adequate protein and carbohydrate at both breakfast and lunch, as suggested in this book, you will have more energy to perform throughout the day. Furthermore, you will have the protein you need to build or maintain muscle. Often, patients who skip meals lose so much muscle that they feel weak throughout the day. (And as we'll see later in this chapter, lost muscle also means a reduced rate of calorie burning.) If you lose weight in a healthy way, you will find that you have more energy than ever, and you will feel lighter and stronger.

Staying Healthy and Living Longer

Being overfat is not just socially undesirable, but can affect how long you live and how healthy you will be during that lifetime. A study by the American Cancer Society, which looked at over 750,000 individuals, showed that being overfat increases one's risk of developing cancer of the breast, colon, prostate, uterus, kidney, and gallbladder. The American Heart Association recently upgraded obesity from a contributing factor to a major risk factor for heart disease, comparable with high blood pressure, smoking, high cholesterol, or diabetes. The American Diabetes Association recognizes the impact of increased body fat on diabetes. Diabetes is a pretty common disease, affecting at least 16 million Americans. It can result in kidney failure, blindness, heart attack, and premature death. Over 80 percent of all diabetics are overfat. If these people simply lost weight, in some cases their diabetes would become undetectable if caught early. In other cases, it would remain detectable but would be easier to control. Similarly, many patients with so-called essential mild high blood pressure (the word "essential" means doctors don't know what the cause is) can reduce their blood pressures, sometimes to the normal range, by losing weight.

When I was in medical training, I would ask my supervisors why all my patients had diabetes, high blood pressure, and high cholesterol. They would say, "Common diseases occur commonly. Go back to work!" Now I know that these common diseases occur commonly because they often have a very common cause—obesity!

A recent study by a large health maintenance organization in northern California showed that 7 percent of their total health care costs were associated with obesity or excess body fat. So being overfat is serious business. Conquering your bad eating, exercise, and stress habits can pay great dividends of longevity and a better quality of life.

GETTING YOUR BODY FAT UNDER CONTROL: WHY CAN'T I DO THIS?

Some people seem to be able to eat whatever they want and not gain weight, while other people look at food and gain several pounds. The difference, as we've seen, lies in genetics. Our genes are 50,000 years old. We have only had a surplus of food for the last 100 years, so our genes have not had a chance to evolve to the diet we have now. There were no fast food restaurants, twenty-four-hour markets, or even refined sugars 50,000 years ago. There was a shortage of food, and being able to go without eating was a real advantage. The thermostat that controls our appetites was set in a time of calorie deficiency, yet we now live in a time of calorie excess. As a result, one of every two to three Americans is genetically predisposed to store fat too efficiently.

Not everyone stores fat in the same place. Let's look at how different people store fat.

Lower Body Fat and Female Hormones

Our society has defined sexiness for women as never being too thin, especially in the lower stomach, hips, and thighs. This is a recent development in human history, dating back to the 1960s. There is no doubt that over the last forty years, the desired weight of American women has fallen way below the average healthy weight. Struggling against your biology is not necessary to be healthy or beautiful. If Marilyn Monroe were alive today, she would be a patient in my clinic complaining that she was 35 pounds overfat!

Lower body fat is called "female" fat, because the female hormones estrogen and progesterone stimulate these fat cells. (Only if men have low male hormone levels can fat accumulate in their hips and thighs.) Puberty is triggered in young women when a critical level of body fat is reached, and this fat is deposited in the hips and thighs as part of normal development. This fat is stored to support future children, since breast milk is 50 percent fat calories. The connection between body fat and reproduction can be seen in women who have eating disorders and anorexia. These women stop having periods and become infertile unless they regain weight, in which case their periods return.

The Venus of Willendorf is a Neanderthal statue that is about 25,000 years old. This is a statue of a stocky woman with large thighs and big breasts, and this view of fat women as sexy persisted throughout much of history for good reason. Stocky women were stronger helpmates on the farm and could bear children in times of famine, when thinner women would become infertile.

Every month, in the last ten days of the menstrual cycle, women often crave fatty, sweet foods due to rising levels of progesterone. This hormone, which prepares the uterus to receive a fertilized egg, causes water retention and an increased appetite, along with headaches, breast tenderness, and irritability. These symptoms are referred to as premenstrual syndrome. If you are trying to control your weight, this last ten days of the month will be a time when you need to get extra sleep, exercise regularly, and pay close attention to what you are going to read in the upcoming chapters. As women age, the progesterone and estrogen effects on their lower body fat accumulate until menopause, when the lower body fat stops growing and in some cases recedes, while upper body fat increases. So your reproductive cycle is closely tied to your appetite and body fat percentage.

If you are fighting your lower-body fat distribution, you are fighting Mother Nature. This is not impossible, but it requires both patience and a strong combination of exercise and diet. Starvation in this situation does more harm than good. You will lose muscle and your metabolism will slow down, while the hormone-programmed fat sticks around. I see many women who look thin, but who have lost muscle and so have a high percentage of fat.

The best approach is to build muscle and lose fat. One counter to the modern "never too thin movement" is the *Sports Illustrated* swimsuit edition. The woman who photographs these models says she selects only fit women with well-developed leg muscles, not the thin, bony models selected by fashion designers. You don't have to have huge, muscular arms if you don't want them. In fact, the largest muscles are in the thighs, where you can replace fat with muscle and improve your health and appearance at the same time.

Upper Body Fat and the King (or Queen) of the Hill

Both men and women can carry fat in the upper body. This pattern of fat distribution is an adaptation to the feast-or-famine situation our ancestors found themselves in. Many people with upper body fat can skip meals without feeling hungry all day, and then can eat all the food in their pantry after dinner. Unfortunately, this fat distribution pattern is associated with an increased risk for diabetes, high blood pressure, heart disease, and breast cancer.

Upper body fat can be associated with an aggressive nature in some people, which in turn has a physical component. For example, many top executives I see are very aggressive. But executives are not the only ones who are kings of the hill. I was driving to work one day and saw a five-man road crew. The foreman's stomach hung out over his belt, which was tightened low over his hips. He stood with his arms folded as he barked out orders to his four thinner, younger helpmates who were doing all the work. Nature provided that foreman with leadership genes for survival. I would not be surprised if his male hormone levels are higher than normal. Women with upper body fat often have higher male hormones than other women.

However, aggression doesn't play well in the small spaces modern humans often find themselves in. If you put a group of male rats or monkeys together, one will emerge as the chief and the others will become submissive. The submissive animals may show reductions in male hormone levels, and in some primate studies equivalents of depression and withdrawal have been observed.

There is a connection between aggression and burn-out depression, the type of condition caused by unrelenting stress. Eating can be a mood elevator or tranquilizer for some people. While some scientists have connected this food-mood relationship to a rise in a brain chemical called serotonin, which they contend increases in response to carbohydrates and sweets, there are probably many variations of this food-mood connection other than sweets. Simply filling up can be a tranquilizer. Humans can develop cravings for many different types of foods other than sweets. I have observed in my practice that patients who reduce "what's eating them" are better able to control what they are eating.

If you have upper body fat, your appetite center is set on overdrive and you will need special help to deal with skipping, starving, and stuffing. If this describes your eating habits, your appetite center may be playing a role in maintaining your body fat. To help you change your behavior, I recommend a wonderful book—*Seven Habits of Highly Effective People* by Steven Covey (see Appendix A). I use his principles in my thinking about behavior and weight loss, and you will learn skills that will help you in other areas of life as well.

Pockets of Fat, Lumps, and Bumps

Beyond these two general types of fat, it is possible for fat to land in special places. Men tend to accumulate breast fat and "love handles," or fat at the sides, after the age of forty. Very commonly, this happens because of changes in hormone levels that occur in men as they age. Some women get a pocket of fat in the lower abdomen after age fifty. These areas of fat are very resistant to weight loss, and if you are really concerned about them, you should consider plastic surgery after you have reached your desired body weight. My general rule is to wait for at least a year after you have controlled your overall body fat and lifestyle before doing this. However, as with all rules, it is made to be broken. I have sometimes found that self-esteem is enhanced when plastic surgery is performed, and this makes weight loss easier to achieve.

EATING BEHAVIORS THAT SABOTAGE
WEIGHT CONTROL

Now that you know where your fat tends to be distributed and why, it's time to learn how your eating behaviors can undermine your attempts to lose weight. By far, the most common eating behavior I see in my clinic is the ability to starve. Those patients with upper body fat can often skip breakfast, skip lunch, and eat the whole refrigerator after dinner. This behavior fits well with the meal replacement approach we will discuss in Chapter 3.

The next most common behavior is the sweet/fat or chocolate "addiction"—people actually have key chains that read "I am a Chocoholic." While not true addictions, which are associated with withdrawal symptoms such as nausea, these strong cravings can feel addictive to the people who experience them.

Boredom, anxiety, love, happiness, and many other emotions can trigger them. These cravings are worse for some women in the ten days before their period, when progesterone levels are high. Cravings for cheese are common among women, and cravings for red meat are common among men.

These cravings are simply strong habits. There is no exact amount of fat we are built to enjoy. As you eat more fat, you get used to its taste-enhancing effect. It also works in reverse; as you get used to low-fat foods you won't like the high-fat foods you used to crave. Breaking habits is not easy. You will need to develop new skills for coping with challenges to your resolve. You will need to use physical activity and stress reduction, and you may want to cultivate a sense of control over your life that can raise your self-esteem.

SETTING YOUR PERSONAL WEIGHT-LOSS TARGET

Now that you have learned why and how you gain weight, it's time to start doing something about it. The amount of weight you want to lose can be determined in one of several ways. First, you can select a healthy percentage of weight loss, such as losing 10 percent of your current body weight. There is some evidence that such small weight losses can benefit your health somewhat, even if you have much more excess weight to lose.

On the other hand, you may wish to lose weight to an optimal percentage of body fat: 15 to 20 percent for men and 22 to 28 percent for women. You can determine your body fat level by having your doctor measure it with a bioelectrical impedance meter. These meters are also available at health clubs, and you can even buy them. The meter sends a very small electric current through your body. Muscle conducts electricity, while fat does not. By measuring the electrical resistance of your body fat, the amount of fat and lean muscle mass can be estimated.

If you don't have access to an impedance meter, you can estimate your target weight from your Body Mass Index (BMI). BMI is your weight divided by your height squared. It is an estimate of body fat, and has been verified by measurements made on thousands of individuals. You can find your BMI by using the chart on pages 28 and 29.

To find your BMI, simply look up your height and then look across to find your weight. At the top of that column you will find the BMI. (If your height does not appear on the chart, see Appendix B to learn how to figure your BMI.) According to the latest guidelines from the National Institutes of Health, body mass index can be used to classify different levels of overweight. A BMI of 25 to 29.9 is considered overweight. A BMI of 30 to 39.9 is considered moderate obesity. A BMI of greater than 40 is considered severe obesity. One estimate of what you should lose is to first find your BMI. Then for your height find that weight that will bring you just below a BMI of 25. This can be your personal weight-loss goal.

How fast will you lose weight? That depends on how many calories your body burns each day. Calorie usage can be measured with what is called a metabolic cart, an apparatus that measures how much oxygen you consume at rest. Since it is not likely that you or your family doctor has a metabolic cart, the next-best predictor of the number of calories you will burn is your lean muscle mass. Each pound of lean mass burns 14 calories per day. So a woman with 100 pounds of lean tissue will burn 1,400 calories per day, while her husband, who has 150 pounds of lean tissue, will burn 2,100 calories per day. (To learn what we mean when we say "calorie," see "What Is a Calorie?" on page 33.)

If you don't have an impedance meter, you can use your BMI and the chart on page 30 to estimate the number of calories you will burn.

If the number of calories per day for your BMI doesn't make sense to you, then you are outside the range of muscle mass that would be average for your BMI. This means that you are particularly strong and athletic (if you have more muscle) or that you may be low in muscle due to repeated dieting efforts in the past.

You can use the chart on page 30 to figure out your weekly weight loss. First, you should simply subtract the number of

Estimate Your Target Body Weight

Body Mass Index

BMI	19	20	21	22	23	24	25	26	27	28	29	30	31	32	33	34	35	36
Height									Weight in Pounds									
4'10"	91	96	100	105	110	115	119	124	129	134	138	143	148	153	158	162	167	172
4'11"	94	99	104	109	114	119	124	128	133	138	143	148	153	158	163	168	173	178
5'0"	97	102	107	112	117	122	127	132	138	143	148	153	158	163	168	174	179	184
5'1"	100	106	111	116	122	127	132	138	143	148	153	158	164	169	174	180	185	190
5'2"	104	109	115	120	126	131	136	142	147	153	158	163	169	175	180	186	191	196
5'3"	107	113	118	124	130	135	141	146	152	158	164	164	169	175	180	186	191	203
5'4"	110	116	122	128	134	140	145	151	157	163	169	175	180	186	192	197	204	209
5'5"	114	120	126	132	138	144	150	156	162	168	174	180	186	192	198	204	210	216
5'6"	116	124	130	136	142	148	155	161	167	173	179	186	192	198	204	210	216	223
5'7"	121	127	134	140	147	153	159	166	172	178	185	191	198	204	211	217	223	230
5'8"	125	132	139	145	152	158	165	172	178	185	191	197	203	210	216	223	230	236
5'9"	128	135	142	149	155	162	169	176	182	189	196	203	209	216	223	230	236	243
5'10"	132	140	147	154	161	168	175	182	189	196	202	209	216	222	229	236	243	250
5'11"	136	143	150	157	164	171	179	186	193	200	208	215	222	229	236	243	250	257
6'0"	140	147	155	162	170	177	185	192	199	207	214	221	228	235	242	250	258	265
6'1"	144	151	158	166	174	181	189	196	204	211	219	227	235	242	250	257	265	272
6'2"	148	155	164	171	179	187	195	203	210	218	225	233	241	249	256	264	272	280
6'3"	152	160	168	176	184	192	200	207	216	224	232	240	248	256	264	272	279	287
6'4"	156	164	172	181	189	197	205	214	222	230	238	246	254	263	271	279	287	295

Clinical guidelines on the identification, evaluation and treatment of overweight and obesity in adults. National Institutes of Health; National Heart, Lung and Blood Institute (1998).

calories in your diet (for example, 1,200 calories) from the estimated total number of calories burned per day (let's say 1,700 calories). If the difference, as in this example, is 500 calories per day, you will lose 1 pound per week, or 4 pounds a month. If the difference is 1,000 calories, you will lose 2 pounds per week or 8 pounds per month. This is only an estimate and will depend on how well you follow your plan.

Estimate Your Target Body Weight

Body Mass Index

BMI	37	38	39	40	41	42	43	44	45	46	47	48	49	50	51	52	53	54
Height								Weight in Pounds										
4'10"	177	181	186	191	196	201	205	210	215	220	224	229	234	239	244	248	253	258
4'11"	183	188	193	198	203	208	212	217	222	227	232	237	242	247	252	257	262	267
5'0"	189	194	199	204	209	215	220	225	230	235	240	245	250	255	261	266	271	276
5'1"	195	201	206	211	217	222	227	232	238	243	248	254	259	264	269	275	280	285
5'2"	202	207	213	218	224	229	235	240	246	251	256	262	267	273	278	284	289	295
5'3"	208	214	220	225	231	237	242	248	254	259	265	270	278	282	287	293	299	304
5'4"	215	221	227	232	238	244	250	256	262	267	273	279	285	291	296	302	308	314
5'5"	222	228	234	240	246	252	258	264	270	276	282	288	294	300	306	312	318	324
5'6"	229	235	241	247	253	260	266	272	278	284	291	297	303	309	315	322	328	334
5'7"	236	242	249	255	261	268	274	280	287	293	299	306	312	319	325	331	338	334
5'8"	243	249	256	262	269	276	282	289	295	302	308	315	322	328	335	341	348	354
5'9"	250	257	263	270	277	284	291	297	304	311	318	324	331	338	345	351	358	365
5'10"	257	264	271	278	285	292	299	306	313	320	327	334	341	348	355	362	369	376
5'11"	265	272	279	286	293	301	308	315	322	329	338	343	351	358	365	372	379	386
6'0"	272	279	287	294	302	309	316	324	331	338	346	353	361	368	375	383	390	397
6'1"	280	288	295	302	310	318	325	333	340	348	355	363	371	378	386	393	401	408
6'2"	287	295	303	311	319	326	334	342	350	358	365	373	381	389	396	404	412	420
6'3"	295	303	311	319	327	335	343	351	359	367	375	383	391	399	407	415	423	431
6'4"	304	312	320	328	336	344	353	361	369	377	385	394	402	410	418	426	435	443

You will be able to tell whether your weight tends to yo-yo up and down with each new diet (high metabolism) or if you simply have a hard time losing any weight with a diet (low metabolism). What does it mean to have a high or low metabolism? The amount of weight you gain or lose depends on how much energy you are burning at any one time. This is called "metabolism." It is made up of many different types of energy

Estimated Rate of Daily Calorie Burning

BMI	Women	Men
25	1,200–1,400	1,700–1,800
26	1,250–1,450	1,730–1,830
27	1,350–1,550	1,760–1,860
28	1,400–1,600	1,800–1,900
29	1,430–1,630	1,830–1,930
30	1,460–1,660	1,850–1,950
31	1,490–1,690	1,880–1,980
32	1,520–1,720	1,900–2,000
33	1,550–1,750	1,950–2,050
34	1,580–1,780	2,000–2,100
35	1,600–1,800	2,050–2,150
36	1,630–1,830	2,100–2,200
37	1,650–1,850	2,150–2,250
38	1,680–1,880	2,200–2,300
39	1,700–1,900	2,250–2,350
40	1,750–1,950	2,300–2,400

Adapted from Mifflin, Mark D., St Jeor S, Hill LA, Scott BJ, Daugherty SA, Koh YO. A new predictive equation for resting energy expenditure in healthy individuals. *American Journal of Clinical Nutrition* 51:241–247 (1990).

burning. The energy you need to just sit and read this book is called "resting metabolic rate," or RMR. This is about 75 percent of the energy you burn each day, with the remaining 25 percent coming from the energy required to digest your food and to exercise. The main factor that determines the number of calories you burn at rest is your lean body mass. This is everything in your body other than your fat tissue. The liver, the digestive system, the brain, and the skeletal muscles all contribute to RMR, and each of these tissues burns lots of energy even at rest. As we've seen, one way to estimate RMR is to multiply lean body mass (preferably measured with an impedance meter), by fourteen, or you can use your BMI and the chart above. If you burn 2,500 calories per day, you are probably a yo-yo dieter who can lose weight with almost any diet. If you burn only 1,100 calories per day, you probably have a lot of trouble losing weight on any diet. Estimating your metabolism helps you to estimate how much weight you will lose on any number of calories, and how many calories you will be able to eat over the long haul to maintain your weight.

Having realistic expectations of what your weight should be and how quickly you can reasonably attain this goal is critical to being able to plan your personal Resolution Diet.

YOUR HABITS AND HOW TO CHANGE THEM

There are stages you will go through in changing your habits. Researchers Prochaska and DiClemente have outlined these stages by studying smokers who stopped smoking successfully on their own, as compared with those in treatment programs. All smokers identified a certain sequence of changes that they cycled through in their attempts to quit smoking:

1. Precontemplation: you are not intending to make any change in the near future.
2. Contemplation: you are considering making a change, but have not yet made a firm commitment to change.
3. Preparation: you are committed to changing your behavior in the next thirty days, but have not yet begun to change.
4. Action: you are successfully changing your behavior.
5. Maintenance: your behavior change has been sustained for six months.

Relapse terminates either the maintenance stage or the action stage, forcing you to go back through the other stages.

Is all this talk about psychology important? Yes, because it makes no sense for me to give you action-oriented advice if you are in the precontemplation stage, when you have no intention of changing. It also makes no sense to give you action-oriented advice if you have already made changes and are now in the maintenance stage. You must identify which stage you are in. Then you can find the right part of the book to use for yourself. If you are in the precontemplation stage, just read through the book from cover to cover, and it may get you ready to change. If you have successfully changed your diet, you may wish to skip to the chapter on relapse prevention (Chapter 8) or you may want more background on educating your palate (Chapter 5).

If these stages don't fit perfectly, don't worry. Changing your diet is much more complicated than stopping smoking. You may be at a precontemplation phase for adding fiber and at a maintenance stage for changing dietary fat intake. It is best to look at this as a general model that can help you identify when you are ready for inspiration, commitment, resolute behavior, or relapse prevention.

You may also change your stages as you read and reread this book. Using the profile at the end of the chapter can help you both keep track of where you are and integrate this behavior information with other information on your physiology, family history, and nutrition to create your personal Resolution Diet. You will want to periodically review this information to see if your answers change.

I have written this book to put together the knowledge, attitudes, and behavior message into a single program. As we progress, you may find you don't agree with a piece of information. If this is the case, I want you to modify it to meet your own needs. You will have the opportunity to do this throughout the book. There is no absolute truth when it comes to human behavior. When I am seeing patients in clinic, I change what I do as I move from room to room to fit the particular patient I am seeing. This book presents a plan that can be tailored to fit your situation.

Since I cannot see you in person as you read this, you will have to help me to shape this program for you. It is also important that you make the right promise to yourself. I once overheard a professor at a cocktail party say, "This New Year's I made a

What Is a Calorie?

When it comes to weight loss, everyone talks about calories. But what is a calorie, exactly?

A calorie is a measure of the amount of energy given off when a certain amount of food is burned. Individual calories represent tiny amounts of energy, though, so it is easier to talk about food energy in terms of kilocalories—1,000 calories taken together. So when we say that a cookie contains 60 "calories," we really mean that it contains 60 "Calories," or 60,000 little calories. To keep things simple, this book uses the term "calories." Just remember that what we call "calories" are really kilocalories, or "Calories."

resolution I knew I could keep. I decided to gain 2 pounds!" While I am not suggesting that you make that resolution, what goal is realistic and right for you?

In the next chapter, I will explain which foods and thoughts are keeping you from losing weight successfully. I will also teach you about the Trigger Food Strategy, which will start you on the road to healthy eating.

Your Readiness-to-Change
PROFILE

Answer the following ten questions to find out how ready you
are to change.

FAMILY/PERSONAL HISTORY FACTORS

1. Which individuals are/were overfat in your family?
   - ☐ Mother   ☐ Father   ☐ Brothers
   - ☐ Sisters   ☐ Aunts   ☐ Uncles

2. When did you start to accumulate excess body fat?
   - ☐ Childhood ☐ Adolescence ☐ Adult ☐ After pregnancy

3. Where is your body fat located?
   - ☐ Upper body ☐ Lower body ☐ Other (where): _____

4. If you have dieted before, which best characterized your
   weight loss?
   - ☐ Lost weight easily but regained (yo-yo)
   - ☐ Lost weight but less than I should have because I didn't
     follow diet
   - ☐ Followed diet carefully but couldn't lose
   - ☐ Didn't follow diet and couldn't lose

PERSONALITY/BEHAVIOR FACTORS

5. Why do you want to lose weight?
   - ☐ Cosmetic concerns
   - ☐ Low-energy concerns
   - ☐ Health concerns

6. Which eating behavior best characterizes your habits?

☐ Meal skipper   ☐ Bread binger   ☐ Cheese lover

☐ Stress eater   ☐ Chocoholic   ☐ Ice cream addict

☐ Chronic dieter   ☐ Meat lover

7. How strong is your desire to lose weight this time, on a scale of 1 to 10, with 1 being the lowest? (circle one)

1   2   3   4   5   6   7   8   9   10

8. How do your rate your chance of success this time, on a scale of 1 to 10, with 1 being the lowest? (circle one)

1   2   3   4   5   6   7   8   9   10

9. At this point in time, what is your overall stage for changing your behavior? (Note changes in stage as they occur.)

	Date	Date	Date	Date
Precontemplation	____	____	____	____
Contemplation	____	____	____	____
Preparation	____	____	____	____
Action	____	____	____	____
Maintenance	____	____	____	____
Relapse	____	____	____	____

SETTING YOUR WEIGHT-LOSS GOAL

10. What is your personal weight-loss goal?

☐ 10 lb.   ☐ 20 lb.   ☐ 30 lb.

☐ 40 lb.   ☐ 50 lb.   ☐ More than 50 lb.

Chapter 3

The Trigger Food Strategy

The key to getting control of your eating habits is learning to enjoy healthy foods that taste great because they excite your taste buds without relying on hidden fat, sugar, and salt. Food-industry advertising is designed to appeal to your emotions. The Resolution Diet is designed to appeal to your common sense without depriving your taste buds.

This chapter will give you my simple Trigger Food Strategy to get you started on your new way of eating. This chapter and Chapter 4 are meant to be read together, because once you are able to employ the Trigger Food Strategy, you will learn in Chapter 4 how to finally take charge of your eating habits using meal replacements and portion-controlled foods. In the very first week that you cut your calorie intake, you will lose some weight. Though this weight won't be all fat, you will feel more confident and comfortable about your new program. Your enthusiasm is always high at the start of something new, so I want to make it simple for you to achieve as much as possible in the first several weeks.

To help you achieve this initial weight loss, I will first explain why the way food is advertised and sold in this country can lead you to lose control of your eating habits. I will outline my

Trigger Food Strategy for getting a hold of your diet. This involves avoiding certain foods, such as pizza, and substituting other foods with similar tastes, such as pasta with tomato sauce. This will allow you to organize your eating patterns, which will give you the best chance of losing weight right off the bat.

My goal in this chapter is to give you a game plan that will show you where to put your early efforts. The following chapters will give you behavior-modification and additional nutritional tools that will allow you to change the way you eat permanently. As in Chapter 2, be sure to fill out the profile at the end of this chapter.

WHO IS IN CONTROL?

The pressure to eat is all around us. We eat food not only to satisfy physical hunger but also for its entertainment value. Eating certain foods in certain settings is made attractive in advertising messages that bombard us every day, in the same ways we are sold on habits such as beer drinking or smoking. (You will notice that someone smoking a cigarette is usually in some appealing situation connected to wealth, attractiveness, or happiness.) Advertising is applied psychology, and your eating habits are being targeted by a serious and efficient business.

Your attitudes towards food and comfort, soothing, and nurturing come from food promotion by the advertising industry. Every time you buy the foods being advertised, you are giving the advertisers the result they expect. If you were to tell the food industry you wanted fat-free foods, they would oblige. In fact, they have obliged with over a thousand fat-free foods in the last ten years. Now manufacturers are putting the fat back into some fat-free cookies, because consumers have said they want better taste more than they want less fat. Yes, this is a food democracy, and you are being represented by millions of average citizens whose spending habits have created a food environment that represents their desires in the following order: taste, cost, convenience, and—in a distant fourth place—health.

Come on an imaginary trip to a typical cafeteria line with me and you will see how hard it can be to get a healthy low-fat meal. You pick up a tray and peer through the glass panel to see the salads. You have a choice of coleslaw made with mayonnaise, an iceberg lettuce-and-tomato salad drowning in Thousand Island or bleu cheese dressing, or a carrot-and-raisin salad made with mayonnaise. Moving on to main dish, you have a choice of lasagna made with cheese swimming in oil, crispy fried chicken with extra oil, or fried fish sticks with 21 grams of fat in six pieces. The vegetables are blanched and overcooked, smothered in tasteless juice with no spices added. There are also mashed potatoes blended with butter and served with gravy, or there is buttered rice and mushrooms. The dessert is either a tapioca pudding, apple pie, devil's food cake, or canned fruit in sugary syrup. By eating this cuisine, you are bound to get between 35 and 50 percent of your calories from fat, and many more calories than you have the time to burn through exercise.

Fast foods are among the best advertised foods. If you choose a fast food restaurant for reasons of convenience or price, you could have a double-hamburger sandwich, fries, and shake, and get 1,200 calories and 49 grams of fat. According to *The New York Times*, McDonald's opens three new restaurants every day, and its corporate goal is to open a restaurant no more than four minutes from any consumer. Seven percent of all Americans eat at McDonald's on a given day. And that is only one fast food chain.

In this toxic food environment, you need a simple strategy to get off the high-calorie merry-go-round. The old idea that you can somehow restrain yourself from eating what you enjoy is hogwash. In fact, dietary restraint can be measured using a special questionnaire developed by Dr. Albert Stunkard and his colleagues at the University of Pennsylvania. Research has shown that restrained eaters are under greater mental stress than individuals who are not restrained. If you have tried dieting by eating smaller portions of the types of foods we just passed in the imaginary cafeteria, then you have suffered from this stress and frustration.

It is one of the myths of dieting that you can consistently choose smaller portions of all the foods we eat and lose weight over the long term. You will not eat a healthy diet, let alone lose weight, if you choose this old-fashioned approach. Life is about enjoyment, not denial.

THE TRIGGER FOOD STRATEGY

The first step in the Resolution Diet is learning to identify and minimize eating certain foods that may be keeping you from losing weight. I call these "trigger foods." These foods have been developed to sell very well. They taste fatty or sweet (or both). They carry lots of calories per bite, or they are the kinds of foods that undermine portion control. Often, with these foods, you can't eat just one!

First, let's look at why trigger foods appeal to you. Then I'll show you how to eliminate these high-calorie foods from your diet.

Why We Love Trigger Foods

Why are trigger foods so appealing? Your taste buds are naturally drawn to sweet, fatty foods. Since ancient times, humans were often without adequate calories of any kind. As a result, our genes drive us to seek out such foods.

Ancient humans (when they could) would fill up on high-fiber, sweet-tasting foods that would provide lots of nutrition with relatively few calories per bite. Today the trigger foods often deliver a sweet taste without the healthy nutrition of their ancient counterparts. Animals were a small part of the ancient diet, and the animals had very little fat when compared with modern domesticated animals. The animal products on the trigger-food list deliver unbelievable amounts of calories and fat in each portion.

Our bodies haven't had much time to adjust to a low-fiber, high-calorie world. There has been refined sugar in the human diet only since A.D. 1600. Refined sugar, which is now in overabundance, triggers the release of insulin from the pancreas, promoting fat storage. Modern fat and oil processing is at most a hundred years old, and cooking oils were not a part of the American diet at present levels until the 1950s. Also, the nature of the oils we eat has changed. We now eat a diet in which the oils from processed foods, such as oils from corn, safflower, cottonseed, and soybeans, are far more plentiful than those oils found in fish, flaxseed, and olives, which were important parts of the ancient diet. This overwhelming excess of processed fats leads to the production of inflammatory substances that promote cancer and accelerate aging.

So our diet is now polluted with extra fat and refined sugar. Are these evil foods? No! It is how they are used that is the key to the situation. These substances are used to sell food based on taste, cost, and convenience. They provide the cheapest way to enhance taste.

The large profits reaped by the food industry make food labeling a political battleground. The industry and its lobbyists, in an attempt to meet consumer demand, try to influence government policies on nutrition, and the public health, represented by a small number of industry, government, academic, and health advocate communities, often suffers as a result. For example, nonfat margarine can be called ultra-fat-free and still derive 100 percent of its calories from fat. Similarly, some nonfat cheeses aren't really nonfat. It's just that according to the current labeling laws, if a food has less than 0.5 gram of fat per serving, the fat count can be rounded down to zero. (It's the only time in mathematics you can do this.) Or diglycerides, which are produced when the body digests fats called triglycerides, can be added to fat-free baked goods without being labeled as fats. I could give you endless examples of how the food industry influences government food policy and food labeling. (For more information on labeling, see the next page.)

How to Read a Nutrition Label

Nutrition Facts

Serving Size ½ cup (114 g)
Servings Per Container 4

Amount Per Serving

Calories 90   Calories from Fat 30

	% Daily Value*
Total Fat 3g	5%
Saturated Fat 0g	0%
Cholesterol 0mg	0%
Sodium 300mg	13%
Total Carbohydrate 13g	4%
Dietary Fiber 3g	12%
Sugars 3g	
Protein 3g	

Vitamin A 80% • Vitamin C 60% • Calcium 4% • Iron 4%

*Percent Daily Values are based on a 2,000 calorie diet. Your Daily Values may be higher or lower depending on your calorie needs:

Nutrient		2,000 Calories	2,500 Calories
Total Fat	Less than	65g	80g
Sat Fat	Less than	20g	25g
Cholesterol	Less than	300mg	300mg
Sodium	Less than	2,400mg	2,400mg
Total Carbohydrate		300g	375g
Fiber		25g	30g

Calories per gram:
Fat 9 • Carbohydrates 4 • Protein 4

and multiply by 100. For a calories-from-fat value of 30, you would get:

$30 \div 90 = .33 \times 100 = 33\%$ calories

Total Fat. To get the number of calories obtained from fat, multiply the grams by nine.

Total Carbohydrate. This includes added refined sugar, natural sugars (such as lactose in milk), and starches found in many food products.

Dietary Fiber. Aim for at least 25 to 35 grams per day.

Sugar. Realize that this number doesn't discriminate between natural fruit sugars and milk sugars, and refined sugars.

Protein. This includes protein from either animal or vegetable sources.

% Daily Value. These percentages are based on estimates for someone eating a 2,000-calorie diet. These values may not apply to you.

Vitamins and Minerals. Check this line to see the percentage of the recommended intakes of specific vitamins and minerals that this food provides. This is only a rough guide.

Footnotes. These general guidelines are based on calorie intakes that may not apply to you.

Serving Size. Be sure to compare the listed serving size with what you call a serving.

Calories. Compare the calories per serving to your meal plan to see how the food fits into your diet.

Calories From Fat. Your diet should get no more than 20% of its calories from fat. To get the percentage of calories from fat, divide the calories-from-fat number by the total calories

The combination of genetic preference for sweet and fatty foods, sophisticated marketing, and government policy has made the high-fat and -sugar trigger foods an overwhelming presence in the American diet. Twenty percent of all Americans eat no vegetables at all each day. In fact, the commonest fruits and vegetables eaten in the United States today are potatoes and tomatoes—that's French fries and ketchup. Like our ancient ancestors, we still crave fat, and we always will. However, you can reduce these cravings to a much more manageable level by becoming aware both of the foods that trigger these cravings and of ways to avoid them.

Learning How to Leave the Trigger Foods Behind

The following strategies will allow you to recognize and avoid the common trigger foods listed on page 44. As shorthand, I sometimes call these the "no-no" foods. This strategy won't work if you feel deprived, so the idea is not only to practice saying "no" to them but to have an immediate substitution strategy ready to go so that you don't feel deprived. Pick the trigger foods that apply to you, and try to make these dietary changes for the rest of your life. For everything I suggest you cut out, there is a suggestion for something else to eat instead. The Hawaiian word for good tasting is "ono." So I say replace the "no-no" foods with "ono" foods.

Nuts and Seeds

Just about all nuts, seeds, and nut butters are high in fat and calories. This includes such favorites as peanuts, macadamia nuts, peanut butter, and pistachios. For example, fourteen peanuts provides 90 calories. If you are having nuts with your drink at a holiday party, you are getting lots of extra calories. You don't have to dive into a pasta salad to retrieve a pine nut, but you should avoid unnecessary snacks made with nuts.

How do you avoid nuts? On planes, I practice saying "tomato juice" just as the stewardess is approaching to ask whether

Those High-Calorie Culprits:
The Trigger Foods

These trigger foods turn you on and get you fat.

Nuts, *including peanuts, macadamia nuts, sunflower seeds, peanut butter*

Cheese and Cheese Pizza, *including nonfat cheese*

Salad Dressings, *including nonfat salad dressing*

Mayonnaise, Margarine, and Butter, *including fat-free spreads*

Red Meat, *including veal, beef, pork, dark-meat poultry, and lamb*

Fatty Fish, *including farm-fed salmon, trout, and catfish*

Ice Cream and Flavored Yogurt, *including nonfat frozen yogurts, and sweetened yogurt desserts*

Cakes, Pastries, and Muffins, *especially if made with vegetable oils, butter, or other fats*

anyone wants honey-roasted peanuts. Have a handful of pretzels, which will cut out half the calories. Or you may not need anything more than the tomato juice, which also provides valuable nutrients. If you want to make a good substitute for nuts at home, try popcorn made in an air popper. There are 45 calories in 3 cups of air-popped popcorn, the least calories per bite of any snack food you can munch. (Watch out for popcorn at the movies, though. There can be over 1,000 calories in a box of oil-popped popcorn.)

Cheese and Pizza

Cheese is very high in fat and calories. Some pizzas are made with olive oil in the crust and cheese on top, so calories add up fast. Avoid both of these common trigger foods.

Pizza is a top-selling food. People risk their lives trying to deliver it in less than thirty minutes. Three slices of pizza, though, can have more than 1,000 calories. You can give up pizza, but it can be a struggle. Give yourself some time and try having a whole wheat pasta with tomato sauce and some shrimp as a substitute. You can have a pizza with no cheese and no added oil in the crust, but it is better to substitute whole wheat pasta whenever you can.

Cheese is a dangerous temptation. A one-ounce slice of regular American cheese has 140 calories. Women often crave cheese, especially in the last two weeks before their menstrual periods. This is part of the hormonal preparation for carrying a baby, in which a woman's body is seeking to deposit some fat. But the cheese habit can be broken. Start by not buying cheese, so that you aren't tempted to add it to a sandwich or snack on it. You can then move onto only eating it at a special event, such as a party. Then buy the grated nonfat cheese to sprinkle on salads or pasta dishes. Ultimately, you are working towards the goal of minimizing your cheese intake, or eliminating it altogether. While cheese is a good source of calcium, I will give you many other calcium sources that don't have the fat and calories of cheese. Contrary to what the dairy industry would have you believe, there is no daily cheese requirement (see page 87).

Nonfat cheese is an outstanding protein source with important uses in healthy prepared dishes. But do not abuse it; eating eight slices of nonfat cheese a day adds 640 calories to your diet.

Salad Dressing

Salads are a healthy part of a good diet. But when you add a high-fat salad dressing made with oil, you add unnecessary calories. (Thousand Island dressing, for example, is made from mayonnaise, ketchup, and relish.) So any salad dressings made with oil, including so-called low-fat salad dressings, are trigger foods. Most regular salad dressings contain about 40 calories per tablespoon, and when you use three times the amount of the low-fat dressings, which contain 14 calories per tablespoon, you end up with the same number of calories.

There are two ways to make a healthy salad. First, switch from creamy, oil-based dressings to vinegar-based dressings. For more flavor, shelve the plain vinegar in favor of balsamic, rice, or wine vinegar. Or try one of the many flavored vinegars on the market, such as raspberry vinegar. Mix in a little mustard to make a Dijon-style dressing.

The second way to make a healthy salad is to use healthy ingredients. Iceberg lettuce and a cucumber slice just won't do. The key here is to make your salad tasty with dark green lettuce, tomatoes, alfalfa sprouts, green and red peppers, and other vegetables (see the list on page 68) so that you don't depend on the dressing to carry the taste. In fact, salads made this way can be used to help you fill up after dinner, if you're still hungry, with very few extra calories compared with most other things you could fill up on.

Butter, Margarine, and Mayonnaise

There are times you may crave butter, a taste Americans have been taught to love. But don't think margarine is the answer. Ultra-fat-free margarine is 100 percent fat. Mayonnaise also falls into this creamy, fatty category.

You can learn to live without all three of these trigger foods. Warm your bread to make it moist, and then try having it plain or with a half of a teaspoonful of fruit jam. At supper, you can try roasted garlic as a spread. When you order toast in a restaurant, ask for high-fiber wheat bread or buns with no added butter or margarine—otherwise they may add a paintbrushful of margarine to your toast. If you are having a meat sandwich, have mustard with no mayonnaise, and add such tasty extras as alfalfa sprouts or sliced cucumber. While you can use fat-free mayonnaise as a stepping stone to giving up mayo entirely, don't fool yourself by stopping there. Your taste buds will never learn to leave mayonnaise behind. Besides, when you eat out, fat-free mayonnaise may not be available, and you will fall back into using regular mayo. Cutting out butter, margarine, and mayonnaise will eliminate a lot of unnecessary fat and calories.

Red Meat and Fatty Fish

One of the easiest places to cut out lots of calories is red meat and fatty fish. Veal, beef, pork, and lamb can add lots of fat and calories to your diet. One fourteen-ounce cut of prime rib has about 1,200 calories and 50 grams of fat. That's all the fat and calories a short woman needs for the entire day. Many Americans have cut way down on red meat intake. If you are trying to lose weight, you ought to be leading the pack! See the list below for smart meat choices.

Picking the Right Meat

	Calories	Fat (grams)
High-Fat Meats (6 oz.)		
Dark-meat chicken (without skin)	388	16
Veal, average cut	397	19
Dark-meat chicken (with skin)	430	26
Pork chop	380	26
Sirloin steak, broiled	458	29
Ground beef, broiled	462	32
Pork loin, braised	532	35
Duck, roasted with skin	573	48
Low-Fat Meats (6 oz.)		
Turkey breast	269	5
Chicken breast (without skin)	276	7

You can cut out meat calories without cutting out meat entirely. As you can see, skinless white meat of chicken or turkey is your best choice. Put anything you want on it. There are great sauces you can cook with, or add steak sauce and pretend it's red meat if you want. Marinate poultry in teriyaki sauce or cover it with mustard. It's your choice—just avoid oil-based marinades.

Even fish can be unhealthy, since salmon, trout, and catfish that are farm-fed are high in fat. If you are in the Northwest or Alaska and order ocean-caught salmon in a restaurant, you will notice a different taste and less fat. See the list below.

Finding the Right Fish

	Calories	Fat (grams)
High-Fat Fish (8 oz.)		
Farmed salmon, broiled	420	21
Fish, fried	462	21
Fast food fish filet deluxe sandwich	560	28
Catfish, breaded, fried	517	31
Shrimp, fried	594	30
Tuna salad sandwich with mayo	720	43
Fried seafood combo	554	28
Low-Fat Fish (8 oz.)		
Fin fish, broiled	280	7
(cod, haddock, halibut, flounder)		
Scallops, broiled or grilled (6 oz.)	200	4
Shrimp, cocktail	300	3
Lobster, steamed	222	1.4
Crab, steamed	231	4
Tuna, canned in water	309	5

If fish is on the menu, substitute halibut, swordfish, canned white tuna packed in water, sea bass, orange roughy, red snapper, or whitefish. Shrimp, scallops, lobster and crab are low in fat. So go ahead and enjoy these shellfish, just as long as they are not breaded, sautéed, or deep fried.

Portion size is also important when adding meat or fish to your menu. A three-ounce portion is about the size of the palm of your hand, and you should have one or two of these with dinner and one at lunch (for 1,200 and 1,500 calorie a day meal plans on pages 72 and 73). This will provide you with the portions recommended by the United States Department of Agriculture. Most Americans overshoot by eating nine- to fourteen-ounce portions of meat at a typical restaurant or steak house.

Frozen Yogurt and Ice Cream

We are conditioned to love ice cream. I remember the fairy tale of the young prince who would marry only the woman who would bring him the most delicious dish possible. None of the dishes he tasted pleased him until one candidate for princess brought gravy and ice cream. He thought this was the greatest dish ever and married the princess. They supposedly lived happily ever after, but I'm not sure the prince didn't turn into an overweight middle-aged monarch with a high cholesterol level!

The story of yogurt is much the same. Eaten traditionally as a slightly sour dairy dish in Europe, it only began to sell well in this country when it was flavored to taste like ice cream. Some yogurts available today contain up to 85 percent of calories as refined sugar, and many fat-free yogurts (and ice creams) still add extra calories as sugar while providing too little protein. If you really like yogurt, keep your eyes open for healthy yogurts with live cultures (it will say so on the container), since the special bacterial cultures in yogurt can be healthy for your digestive tract. Get the plain variety, and add fresh fruit if you want a touch of sweetness.

Cakes, Pastries, and Muffins

Cakes and cookies are often made with lots of hidden fat. When I was a kid, I would have to drink a glass of milk to help me chew the tough oatmeal cookies I would get at school. Today, the oatmeal cookies have enough oil in them to give them a puttylike texture. When you chew them, they hardly resist your bite at all. Unfortunately, when combined with chocolate chips and heated, these high-fat cookies become irresistible. In a similar manner, cakes were dry until cooking oil was added. You will often see what looks like a healthy oat bran muffin, only to learn that it is full of extra hidden fat calories as cooking oil. Finally, that croissant you wanted to eat at the coffee shop has an unbelievable 11 grams of fat.

While some of the foods in this category seem to be more obvious sources of sweet and fat than others, you should avoid them all whenever possible. If you have to have a cookie, there are some low-fat choices that are better. I have listed them below, but you should also consider having some fruit, which will substitute great taste and more nutrition for the sweetness of a cookie or a piece of cake (you will find fruits and vegetables listed on page 68).

Picking the Lower-Fat Snacks

	Calories	Fat (grams)
High-Fat Cakes and Pastries		
Oatmeal raisin cookies (4)	235	8
Butter cookies (10 small)	229	9
Danish (1 small)	161	9
Peanut butter cookies (4)	200	10
Chocolate chip cookie, large	190	11
Oreo cookies (6)	300	12
Doughnut, glazed old-fashioned	310	18
Cream puff, with custard filling	303	18
Low-Fat Choices		
Animal crackers (5)	56	1
Graham crackers (6)	180	3

Overcoming Negative Thoughts to Launch Your Trigger Food Strategy

You are now in the initial phase of your Resolution Diet. You have learned a lot of useful information—how to set a weight-loss goal, why you eat the way you do, how to avoid trigger foods. But a great deal of scientific research indicates that information alone will not change your behavior. You need to use this information before you can change. But how? The simple answer you sometimes hear is "Just do it!"

In truth, behavior change is just not that easy. The same traits that make it possible for humans to learn new things through repetition also make all of us stick to old behaviors long after we know that they don't make sense. While smoking and alcoholism are habits that are driven by both a true physical addiction and a psychological dependence, food habits have some of the same characteristics. You hear people say that they are "junk food junkies" or "chocoholics." Many of my patients feel just as trapped in their habits as if they were actually addicted.

One of the keys to my work with patients has been my belief in combining nutrition and behavior messages into action items. However, I sometimes have to deal with patients who are blocked by negative thinking and other self-imposed barriers to change. After I have given my initial advice to a patient, I can see when they are hesitant to change based on their body language and things they may say. You may feel the same way they do. In this section I will outline some of the messages that I use with my patients to reinforce my call to action.

Make a Minimum Effort for a Maximum Impact

One key to changing your diet is to expend your efforts on the changes that will have the maximum impact. For example, if you eat red meat now, you are taking in up to 1,200 calories in a single slice of prime rib. By changing this one habit, you will make a significant impact on your overall diet. Maybe your trigger food is cheese. Then get ready to dump a whole bunch of calories and fat out of your diet by eliminating cheese. It will help to note the "trigger behavior," such as anger or loneliness, that is associated in your case with a particular trigger food, and to find ways to disconnect the behavior from the food. Also, many diets become tiresome because there is so much you have to remember about exchange lists and portions. My message is: don't sweat the small stuff. Take what you learn in this book and apply it to the areas where you need help most.

Change Your Negative Thoughts to Positive Thoughts

You may have tried other diets and failed. You may be someone who just can't stick with a plan. The first step is to believe that you can succeed by changing negative into positive thoughts. Let's look at some examples of negative thoughts you can change into positive thoughts.

"I can't ever lose weight on diets. My metabolism must be too low." You will learn to accept that while you may lose weight more slowly than taller or more muscular people, you will still be able to lose weight.

"I know what to eat already, I just don't do it." The problem may not be what you're eating, but what's eating you. No diet can deal with stress eating, but you can learn how to reduce stress (see Chapter 7) and separate it from your eating patterns.

"I can lose weight on any diet, but I just can't stick with it. I get bored." You are probably blessed with a fast metabolism that allows you to lose weight on almost any diet. In fact, you are like a yo-yo, with your weight going up every time you go off your "diet." You will learn to develop your own diet for a lifetime. By continually refining your diet and lifestyle to maximize taste and variety, you won't get bored.

"Why should I believe that your diet is different, anyway?" You need to give this plan a chance. You may be more comfortable with the idea of failing in advance. That way, there is no risk that it could be your responsibility to eat properly. If you are always looking outside yourself for reasons why things don't

work for you, you should reexamine your behaviors in other areas of your life.

Become Aware of Unconscious Eating

You would be surprised at how often I am sitting with someone who is eating unconsciously. Whether it is taco chips in a Mexican restaurant, popcorn in a movie theater, or peanuts on an airplane, many of us eat without thinking. You are not hungry, you are not craving food, but you have some level of tension in your life and the food is there—so you eat it. To break this cycle, you must become aware of your unconscious eating by becoming aware of the events that lead to mindless munching. Do you finish the leftovers while clearing the dishes? Do you always eat in front of the television? Find the habits that set the stage for unconscious eating, and make some conscious changes. Keep a diary for a day or two of when and where you eat. Then put up a sign that warns you not to eat in the kitchen. Or go for a walk after dinner to fill that high-risk time when snacking happens. Or clear the pantry of your favorite "TV foods." You might be surprised at how much easier it is to lose weight when you actually think about what you are eating.

Don't Try To Be Perfect—80 or 90 Percent Is OK

If you try to be perfect, you are setting yourself up for failure. Setting reasonable goals and expecting to goof up once in a while is the best prescription for success. Don't mistake what I am saying here. You know you are off your personal plan when you eat a handful of peanuts. In Chapter 8, I will teach you how to prevent these lapses from leading to your giving up altogether. Right now, you should expect not to be perfect. However, when you do goof up, it's no excuse for quitting. You are still on the plan, but you will need to think about why you went against your resolution, and what you can do to act differently in the future. On the other hand, if it is a special occasion like a birthday or vacation, it is OK to plan to give yourself the day off. Just be sure that there is not a party every week.

Stress eaters eat when they are happy, sad, lonely, or loved, but rarely when they are simply hungry. If this profile fits you, then watch out for the stress-driven exceptions that come around too frequently. Just don't get down on yourself for not being perfect. No one is.

Work Your Way Towards the Toughest Goals

I had a tough time giving up pizza. It took me two years to consistently be able to avoid this old favorite. Giving up red meat was easier, but going from turkey burgers (made with a mixture of dark and white meat) to white meat of chicken and turkey only took me six months. I want you to know that these behavior changes are tough. Some are tougher than others. Start working on the tough goals today, using my principles of substituting something healthy for your current high-fat favorite. Just don't expect that you will be able to change these permanently overnight.

Resolve to avoid or minimize the trigger foods. Have them memorized, so that when you see them you will run the other way. My greatest successes are with patients who simply follow the trigger food strategy, and who use meal replacements and portion-controlled foods without trying to outsmart me or themselves. You will learn how to do this in the next chapter.

Your Initial Nutrition
PROFILE

Answer the following eleven questions to determine how you can achieve your initial nutrition goals.

FINDING YOUR TRIGGER FOODS

1. Evaluate each of the trigger foods from 1 to 5 (1 being your least favorite, 5 being a great craving).

   _____ Nuts and seeds

   _____ Cheese and pizza

   _____ Salad dressings made with oil

   _____ Butter, margarine, and mayonnaise

   _____ Red meat, including veal, beef, pork, and lamb

   _____ Fatty fish, including salmon, trout, and catfish

   _____ Nonfat yogurt and ice cream

   _____ Cookies, pastries, and cakes

2. What are your own personal trigger foods, including items that are not on the list?

MAKING MINIMUM EFFORTS FOR MAXIMUM CHANGES

3. What are your personal trigger foods and the associated behaviors? (check each that applies and connect the behavior with the trigger)

Trigger foods

☐ Nuts and seeds

☐ Cheese and pizza

☐ Salad dressing

☐ Butter, margarine, mayo

☐ Red meat and fatty fish

☐ Nonfat yogurt and ice cream

☐ Other:_____

Trigger behaviors

☐ Stress/anxiety

☐ Loneliness

☐ Feeling blue

☐ Feeling happy

☐ Anger

☐ Guilt

☐ Other:_____

4. How can you design a strategy to disconnect the trigger behavior and the trigger food?

CHANGING TO A POSITIVE ATTITUDE

5. What are your negative attitudes? (check each that applies below)

☐ I can't lose weight on diets, my metabolism must be too low

☐ I know what to eat already, I just don't do it

☐ I can lose weight on any diet, but I get bored

☐ I don't believe your diet is any different

☐ Other:_____

6. What positive attitudes could you adopt?
   (check each that applies below)

   ☐ I am able to lose weight, but I may lose more slowly than I expect

   ☐ I will be able to follow the diet, if I change my stress eating patterns

   ☐ I can keep from getting bored, if I change my lifestyle so I will always keep developing new goals of diet, exercise, and behavior

   ☐ I will give this diet a chance by going through all the phases, without deciding I am going to fail in advance

   ☐ Other:_____

7. How can you practice self-talk to ingrain your new positive attitude until it is second nature?

UNCONSCIOUS EATING

8. What foods do you binge unconsciously on? (check all that apply)

   ☐ Chips   ☐ Bread   ☐ Peanuts

   ☐ Pretzels   ☐ Cheese   ☐ Cookies or baked goods

   ☐ Other:_____

9. Keep track of the foods you eat unconsciously to determine the triggers. How can you disconnect unconscious eating from the triggering behavior?

CHANGING ATTITUDES

10. What are the problems that can get in your way? (check all that apply)
    ☐ Trying to be perfect
    ☐ Trying to instantly reach all my goals
    ☐ Others?

11. What are the solutions that can help?
    ☐ Aim for 80% to 90% success
    ☐ Approach toughest goals slowly
    ☐ Others?

Chapter 4

Meal Replacements and Portion-Controlled Foods

Y ou are now able to identify both the trigger foods that are keeping you from losing weight and the negative thought processes that go along with those trigger foods. The next step is to get control of your eating habits using meal replacements and portion-controlled meals.

When you try to control the foods you eat, it is hard to know the number of calories you are really eating in any meal. Hidden fats, extra calories, or an extra helping of even "good" foods here and there can really add up. In fact, studies by Dr. Heymsfield at Columbia University demonstrated that dieters usually underestimate their food intake by up to 1,000 calories per day. No wonder you are having so much trouble losing weight! Even if you have eliminated all the trigger foods I mentioned in Chapter 3, you may still be eating large portions on the run, or just eating too many calories to burn off. Skipping meals altogether is definitely not the answer, since that will leave you feeling weak and deprived. Meal replacements and portion-controlled meals give you the security of knowing how many calories you are eating at each meal every day, while providing you with energy, good taste, and healthy nutrition. In this chapter, you will learn how effective the right kind of meal replacement can be in helping you lose weight, especially when combined with portion-controlled meals, fruits, and vegetables into a complete, nutritious meal plan. Meal replacements can help you maintain a healthy diet whenever you don't have time to eat or there is nothing but junk food available. If you ever find yourself slipping back at any time, you can come back to this chapter and refresh your skills in order to regain control of your eating. Use the profile at the end of the chapter to track your progress.

USING MEAL REPLACEMENTS TO CUT CALORIES

How can you cut calories easily and efficiently to reach your goal weight? For most of my patients, eating two meal replacements each day—together with healthy fruits and vegetables, and a healthy portion-controlled meal—is the easiest way to do this. If you have a lot of time and want to prepare and measure the types of foods you will learn about in this book, that's great. You will also lose weight, but it may be more difficult and the rate of loss will be slower. Meal replacements provide a convenient and cost-effective shortcut. A well-designed meal replacement provides enough calories to meet the recommendations of most dietitians and doctors, who believe in healthy weight loss. Meal replacements and portion-controlled foods will make it easier for you to accomplish your weight-loss goals. You may find that these tools remove the anxiety and uncertainty from dieting, and provide the easiest path from where you are now to where you want to be.

Meal replacements can be a great tool to help you achieve your goal of permanent weight loss. Look at it this way. You have twenty-one meals each week (three per day) with maybe seven to fourteen snacks a week. If you can save 3,500 calories a week, or just 500 calories a day, you will lose a pound a week, or fifty pounds a year. If you can use a meal replacement for ten or more meals per week (that's five of seven days), you will make a definite dent in your calorie intake. If you can do this fourteen times a week, you will be getting the maximum possible benefit by replacing breakfast and lunch, and then having a portion-controlled dinner. The amount of weight you will lose with this plan will vary, depending on your metabolism (see Chapter 2) and starting weight.

Weight Control and the Science of Meal Replacements

The basic fact of weight gain and loss is this: In order to lose weight, you must take in fewer calories than you burn. There are two ways for you to reach this goal. You can eat fewer calories by eliminating the trigger foods, and by eating meal replacements and portion-controlled foods, or you can increase the calories you burn through exercise (see Chapter 7). The most efficient way to go about it is to use both of these methods together.

While many diets are based on some supposedly special property of either fat, protein, or carbohydrate, you need to understand that the human body can convert calories between all three basic food types. (To learn exactly what these terms mean, see "Carbohydrate, Protein, and Fat—Defining the Terms" on page 63.) This means that anything you eat—from a cheesecake to a sandwich to a steak—can turn into body fat if it is not burned as fuel.

How does the body process the calories you eat? Remember, calories represent energy. The body stores only 1,200 calories—one day's worth—of energy as carbohydrates, but about 130,000 to 160,000 calories as fat. This would be about 20 slices of sourdough bread versus about 120 fourteen-ounce cuts of prime rib, or less than one day's supply of energy stored as carbohydrate but about eighty days stored as fat. The body is set up this way because carbohydrates are used for short-term energy on a day-to-day basis. While a very small fraction of your stored fat is burned every day, its most important role is to provide most of the calories needed during prolonged periods of starvation. (In fact, I teach my patients that how well their bodies can hang onto fat would determine how long they could survive if lost in the desert.) You also carry about 54,000 calories of protein in your muscles and organs, but this is more than mere energy. This protein is precious because it is part of life-giving processes in the muscles, liver, heart, and immune system. It is not possible to survive if you use more than half your body's protein stores. Therefore, your body conserves protein under starvation conditions by using fat stores.

These differences between what you eat and what you store have important implications. First, you can see that carbohydrate needs to be replenished daily. Protein and fat are vital to survival, which makes the storage of these nutrients critically important. The idea is that since the human body evolved under starvation conditions, it is programmed to retain fat and a relatively small amount of carbohydrate in order to protect protein stores. You are what you eat, but only indirectly. Our bodies can convert carbohydrate, fat, and protein into stored fat calories. Of course, there are differences between individuals. I have known patients who would be able to lose weight easily and get away with pretty poor eating habits. On the other hand, I have had patients who eat very well and cannot lose weight easily. But losing weight with ease or with difficulty has nothing to do with counting proteins or carbs or fat grams. You don't need to force your diet out of balance in order to lose weight. There is only one simple fact you need to remember: *Take in fewer calories than you burn and you will lose weight.* Meal replacements can help you do this while keeping necessary nutrients in balance.

Choosing a Meal Replacement

What are my criteria for choosing a meal replacement? First, it must provide healthy nutrition, including high-quality protein, fiber, minerals, and vitamins. Second, it must taste good, so that you will incorporate into your diet for the long term. Third, it must be affordable and widely available.

Carbohydrate, Protein, and Fat— Defining the Terms

What are carbohydrate, protein, and fat, anyway? These are the basic types of foods you eat for energy. They are all made of basic elements: carbon, hydrogen, and oxygen, and in the case of protein, nitrogen and sometimes sulfur. The differences between them lie in the way these basic elements are put together in terms of chemical structure. Carbohydrates (carbs) are either simple or complex. Simple carbohydrates include sugars such as table sugar, corn syrup (the sweetener used in colas), milk sugar, and fruit sugars. Complex carbohydrates are starches found in cereals and breads, which are digested more slowly than sugars. Carbohydrates are an important source of everyday energy. Proteins are made of simple units called amino acids. There are twenty-one common amino acids, of which thirteen must be obtained from the diet. Protein forms the structure of muscles and other tissues. (This is one reason why protein is an important part of the diet. If you don't eat enough protein, you will lose muscle mass.) Fat is usually found in the body in the form of fatty acids. When three fatty acids are connected to a carbon backbone, the result is called a triglyceride. These triglyceride structures make up 90 percent of the fat we eat and store. Other fats include steroid hormones, cholesterol, bile acids, and specialized fats found in cell walls.

While there are several meal replacements that fit this description, the one I have had the most experience with is Ultra Slim-Fast. I have personally prescribed it for thousands of patients, and I have conducted a study with over 300 participants at six different sites throughout the United States using Ultra Slim-Fast under conditions similar to those under which you might use this product. In this study, published in the *Journal of the American College of Nutrition*, 71 men and 230 women participated in a twelve-week weight-loss program, and then continued to use Ultra Slim-Fast for two years to maintain their weight. Of those who started, 91 percent completed the first twelve weeks of the study, and men lost an average of almost 19 pounds while women lost an average of 14 pounds. Both men and women lost about 7 percent of their body weight. A total of 133 people stayed with the program the full two years, which represents 56 percent of the total group. After two years, men maintained an average weight loss of 14 pounds, and women maintained an average weight loss of 13.6 pounds.

At the University of Ulm in Germany, Dr. Ditschuneit and his colleagues compared the use of two meal replacements (Ultra Slim-Fast) per day with simply trying to count calories (between 1,200 and 1,500 calories per day). The group using meal replacements lost an average of over 15 pounds, while those who simply cut back on food intake lost only 3 pounds on average after twelve weeks. Over the following twenty-four months, the meal replacement group lost an average of an additional 6.6 pounds, or a total of about 20 pounds, using just one meal replacement per day. This study scientifically confirms the important role of meal replacements in weight loss, which I have seen in my own practice over the past twenty years.

Between 1992 and 1997, residents of Pound, Wisconsin were given coupons for free Ultra Slim-Fast to replace an average of one meal per day. Over that five-year period, the participants lost and kept off an average of from 9 to 12 pounds. This occurred at a time when people across the nation gained weight on average. In fact, the mayor of Pound, who himself lost 42 pounds, jokingly suggested changing the name of the town to Ounce, Wisconsin!

All of the above studies show that cutting calories and fat using a meal replacement does lead to sustained weight loss.

At the UCLA Center for Human Nutrition, my colleagues and I continue to study meal replacements for weight loss. Recently, we studied a new meal replacement bar (Ultra Slim-Fast Meal On-The-Go Bar). For those on the go, these bars provide an easy way to eat while controlling calorie intake. This new product serves as a complete meal replacement, providing protein, carbohydrate, and fat. Twenty people in our study lost an average of 15 pounds in twelve weeks at a healthy pace of 1.25 pounds per week.

There are other meal replacement shakes and bars available as well. If the nutritional value is the same and you like the taste, then go for it. However, read the label carefully to ensure that there is adequate fiber, since this is important in having a filling effect in your stomach. And if the cost is outrageous, you won't use it for the long term. So you should either use Ultra Slim-Fast or a meal replacement that is a nutritional equivalent, tastes good, is economical, and is widely available. I encourage you to find the meal replacement that is best for you.

Weight loss with meal replacement shakes or bars is not some sort of magical process. A meal replacement takes the place of skipping a meal, while providing a balance of nutrients designed for weight loss. For example, you could have a meal replacement such as Ultra Slim-Fast instead of a deli-counter tuna sandwich for lunch. The tuna sandwich would have 722 calories, 54 grams of fat, and only some of the essential vitamins and minerals you need every day. The meal replacement would have only 220 calories and 3 grams of fat, along with about one-third of the daily requirement for vitamins and minerals. For calcium, which is important for strong bones, the meal replacement would have about 40 percent of the daily requirement in a single serving. I suggest to my patients that they keep a six-pack of canned shakes in the car in case they miss a meal. It beats pulling into a fast food restaurant on the way home. You can also freeze these shakes and eat them in the form of ice cream.

If you will be having a number of meal replacements a week, you will probably want to give them a little variety. You can create your own variations—just make sure you use noncalorie flavorings. Or you can try these suggestions:

- Almond: $1/4$ teaspoon almond extract in a vanilla shake

- Cappuccino: 1 teaspoon instant coffee in a chocolate shake

- Eggnog: $1/2$ teaspoon rum extract, $1/2$ teaspoon apple pie spice in a vanilla shake

- Mint: $1/2$ teaspoon peppermint extract in a chocolate or vanilla shake

- Pina Colada: 1 teaspoon coconut extract, 1 teaspoon rum extract in a vanilla shake

A product like Ultra Slim-Fast is not meant to be your only source of nutrition. It is not intended to replace all of your eating in any day. It is meant to replace one or two meals each day, and perhaps some snacks.

Using Meal Replacements for Life

Many of my patients find that having a meal replacement once per day, at breakfast or lunch, reminds them to watch themselves the rest of the day and makes up for unexpected lapses in eating behavior that can occur. There is nothing unhealthy about eating a meal replacement every day for life. For example, the Ultra Slim-Fast Shake has from 30 to 35 percent of the daily requirement of twenty-four vitamins and minerals. Many of these vitamins and minerals, such as calcium and folic acid, are some of the most important nutrients for maintaining your health. In order to show you just how the whole diet might look, I have analyzed typical menus for their nutritional contents (see pages 72 and 73) at both 1,200 calories per day and 1,500 calories per day, using either one or two shakes per day plus portion-controlled meals (which are discussed on page 67).

In the nutritional analysis I have provided, there is little difference between the final reported calories eaten on these diets using meal replacements and the advice you would get from any nutrition expert. The difference is that you will actually eat the number of calories listed on a regular basis. Knowing how many calories there are per serving and how large each serving is going to be allows you to control your eating once and for all.

If you find yourself very busy, or for any reason need to go off your weight-loss plan, see if you can have at least one shake or meal replacement bar each day. This way you will continue to lose weight, although at a slower rate. Also remember to use portion-controlled foods, and to avoid the trigger foods as much as possible. You will be surprised at how much progress you make with this plan.

SUPPLEMENTING THE MEAL REPLACEMENT WITH FRUITS AND VEGETABLES

Each meal replacement shake or bar contains the carbohydrate, protein, fiber, calcium, and other vitamins and minerals you need. By supplementing this healthy base with vegetables and fruits, you will increase your intake both of these vital nutrients and of disease-preventing substances that are not available in meal replacements or dietary supplements. The beauty of this approach is that it provides complete nutrition without the fat and calories.

Keep in mind, though, that vegetables and fruits are not "free" foods—they do have calories. For example, 1 cup of starchy vegetables, such as beans or potatoes, can pack in over 200 calories. Just 1/4 cup of dried fruit, such as raisins, has over 100 calories. And, if you eat several bunches of grapes or several handfuls of cherries each day, you can slow or even stop your weight-loss efforts. Freely choose from among the fruits and vegetables on List 1 (page 68) to save calories while still getting a full range of health benefits. Choose only 1 cup per serving of the vegetables on List 2 (page 69). Avoid the fruits on List 3 (page 69) while losing weight, so that you can control your fruit portions more easily. Canned vegetables, while often low in calories, contain less vitamin C, fiber, and other nutrients than their fresh counterparts. Therefore, these are not recommended.

CHOOSING HEALTHY PORTION-CONTROLLED MEALS

At least one meal per day should be made up of traditional foods (avoiding the trigger foods, of course). The secret to controlling weight is controlling portions. Here's a good plan for starters. At lunch, if you don't want a meal replacement, have

List 1. Healthy Fruits and Vegetables

Item	Calories	Fiber (g)
Choose Vegetables From This List:		
¹/₂ cup butternut squash (cooked)	41	1.7
¹/₂ cup carrots (cooked)	35	1.5
¹/₂ cup or 1 small whole tomato (raw)	26	1.6
¹/₂ cup broccoli (cooked)	22	2.0
¹/₂ cup or 6 spears asparagus (cooked)	22	1.8
¹/₂ cup spinach (cooked)	21	2.0
¹/₂ cup cauliflower (cooked)	15	1.4
¹/₂ cup zucchini (cooked)	14	1.3
¹/₂ cup bell peppers (raw)	13	0.8
1 cup romaine lettuce (raw)	8	1.0
Choose Fruits From This List:		
1 medium banana	114	1.8
1 medium pear	98	4.3
1 medium apple (with skin)	81	3.0
1 medium orange	59	2.9
1 medium peach	37	1.4
¹/₂ medium grapefruit	37	0.7
1 medium plum	36	1.0
1 cup blueberries	82	3.3
1 cup raspberries	61	5.8
1 cup cantaloupe	57	1.3
1 cup watermelon	50	0.6
1 cup strawberries	45	3.9

List 2. Starchy Vegetables

Item	Calories Per 1 Cup
Eat 1 cup of these starchy vegetables, or *1 cup brown rice at lunch or dinner*	
Garbanzo beans	269
Black beans	241
Lentils	231
Kidney beans	225
Baked potato (1 7-oz.potato)	220
Lima Beans	217
Yellow Corn	178
Yams (cubed)	158
Peas	134

List 3. Fruits to Avoid

Item	Calories Per 1 Cup
Dried fruit	450
Cherries (20)	98
Grapes (20)	82
Canned fruit	60–188

a sandwich made with 3 ounces of skinless chicken or turkey breast, or tuna fish, on two slices of high-fiber bread. In addition, have 2 cups of dark, leafy salad greens with seasoned vinegar and a piece of fruit (such as an apple or a pear) for some healthy and filling fiber. Or have a salad with chicken or fish and a piece of fruit.

For dinner, have 3 ounces of skinless chicken or turkey breast, fish, or shrimp. Three ounces is about the size of the palm of your hand or a deck of cards. So, you can have one palm's worth. Have 1 cup of brown rice, whole wheat pasta, or starchy vegetables (such as corn, beans, or potatoes). You can round out your meal with 2 cups of steamed vegetables (from the vegetable list on page 68) and a large green salad. You could also have cut-up fruit for dessert and still come away eating about 500 calories.

If it is easier for you, just warm up a frozen portion-controlled meal in the microwave or oven. Most supermarkets carry a variety of brands, such as Healthy Choice, Lean Cuisine, and Weight Watchers. Just be sure that you are choosing an entrée with less than 300 calories and less than 25 percent fat. Stay away from red meat and cheese-heavy dishes, since these are the tastes you are trying to get away from. Add a large green salad to complete your meal.

When you are having two meal replacement shakes or bars and one meal a day, you can have the dinner suggested above at lunch time and then have the meal replacement, fruit, and vegetable at night if you wish. That way, you can enjoy the flexibility of eating lunch with friends and still save calories at night. If you are having trouble with nighttime stress-eating, try having air-popped popcorn, which only has 45 calories per 3 cups. Remember to keep a ready-to-drink meal replacement shake on hand, so that you can have one whenever you are tempted to skip a meal or if you find yourself someplace where you cannot get a healthy meal—your car, an airport, a shopping mall, and so forth.

This basic meal plan provides about 1,200 calories a day. If you normally burn about 2,000 calories per day, you will lose about 6 pounds per month on this type of plan. If you burn only 1,500 calories per day, you may only lose 2 or 3 pounds per month. If you exercise (see Chapter 7), you can increase the amounts of weight lost. You won't be living on 1,200 calories, but on the 1,200 dietary calories and 300 to 800 or more calories from your stored fat. The longer you can stay on this plan, the more quickly you will reach your weight goal.

If you are one of those people who can skip breakfast, skip lunch, and then eat the whole refrigerator for dinner, I recommend that you start by using a meal replacement plan, using healthy meal-replacement shakes or bars such as Ultra Slim-Fast for breakfast and lunch, and a portion-controlled meal for dinner. This strategy will lead to success for most dieters right off the bat.

CHOOSING YOUR MEAL REPLACEMENT PLANS

Two plans (with nutritional analyses for typical choices) are outlined on the following two pages: one provides about 1,200 calories a day, the other about 1,500 calories a day. (See Appendix C for detailed meal choices.) Since the choices you make may vary, these plans are meant to guide you to approximate calorie levels. However, the exact amounts of calories and nutrients may vary slightly. In each case, you can make lunch the main meal and have the meal replacement at dinner.

You have learned how to use meal replacements and portion control to help subtract fat and calories from your diet. While you are losing weight, it is important to maintain a difference between the number of calories your body burns and the number of calories in your diet. It is easier to accomplish this goal with a fairly narrow set of food choices, including meal replacements and portion-controlled meals. After you have reached your target weight, you will be able to eat a greater variety and amount of fruits, vegetables, and whole grain foods. But meal replacements and portion-controlled meals will still be useful tools in helping you maintain your new, lower weight for the rest of your life. In the next chapter, you will learn more about eating for a lifetime so that your food choices remain healthy.

A 1,200-CALORIE A DAY PLAN

Stage 1: Two Meal Replacements Per Day

Breakfast: ■ Meal replacement, 1 fruit   *(about 280 calories)*

Lunch: ■ Meal replacement, 1 fruit, 2 cups salad greens with seasoned vinegar   *(about 380 calories)*

PM Snack: ■ 1 fruit, 1 rice cake   *(about 100 calories)*

Dinner: ■ 3 ounces skinless chicken breast, turkey breast, or *(about 435* fish; 1 cup brown rice, whole wheat pasta, or starchy *calories)* vegetable; 2 cups steamed vegetables; 1 fruit; salad

---

Total Calories: 1,195   Total Fiber: 30–35 g
Carbs: 203 g—68% cal.   Fat: 13 g—10% cal.   Protein: 66 g—22% cal.

Stage 2: One or Two Meal Replacements Per Day

Breakfast: ■ Meal replacement, 1 fruit, *or*
(about 280 ■ 1 cup high-fiber cereal with 1 cup fat-free milk,
calories) 1 fruit, *or*

■ 3 egg whites (as little yellow as possible), 1 slice high-fiber bread, 1 fruit

Lunch: ■ Sandwich (3 ounces skinless chicken or turkey
(about 445 breast, or tuna, 2 slices high-fiber bread), 1 fruit,
calories) 2 cups salad greens with seasoned vinegar, *or*

■ 3 ounces sliced chicken, turkey, or tuna; 2 cups salad greens with seasoned vinegar, 1 fruit, *or*

■ Meal replacement, 1 fruit, 2 vegetables

PM Snack: ■ 1 fruit with 1 rice cake   *(about 100 calories)*

Dinner: ■ 3 ounces skinless chicken breast, turkey breast, or
(about 435 fish; 1 cup brown rice, whole wheat pasta, or starchy
calories) vegetable; 2 cups steamed vegetables; 1 fruit; salad

---

Total Calories: 1,260   Total Fiber: 30–35 g
Carbs: 195 g—62% cal.   Fat: 13 g—9% cal.   Protein: 88 g—28% cal.

A 1,500-CALORIE A DAY PLAN

Stage 1: Two Meal Replacements Per Day

Breakfast: ■ Meal replacement, 1 fruit   *(about 280 calories)*

Lunch: ■ Meal replacement, 1 fruit, 2 cups salad greens with seasoned vinegar   *(about 380 calories)*

PM Snack: ■ Meal replacement, 1 fruit, 2 rice cakes   *(about 350 calories)*

Dinner: ■ 6 ounces skinless chicken breast, turkey breast, or
(about 500 fish; 1 cup brown rice, whole wheat pasta, or starchy
calories) vegetable; 2 cups steamed vegetables; 1 fruit; salad

---

Total Calories: 1,510   Total Fiber: 30–35 g
Carbs: 238 g—63% cal.   Fat: 17 g—10% cal.   Protein: 102 g—27% cal.

Stage 2: One or Two Meal Replacements Per Day

Breakfast: ■ Meal replacement, 1 fruit, *or*
(about 280 ■ 1 cup high-fiber cereal with 1 cup fat-free milk,
calories) 1 fruit, *or*

■ 3 egg whites (as little yellow as possible), 1 slice high-fiber bread, 1 fruit

Lunch: ■ Sandwich (3 ounces skinless chicken or turkey
(about 445 breast, or tuna, 2 slices high-fiber bread), 1 fruit,
calories) 2 cups salad greens with seasoned vinegar, *or*

■ 3 ounces sliced chicken, turkey, or tuna; 2 cups salad greens with seasoned vinegar, 1 fruit, *or*

■ Meal replacement, 1 fruit, 2 vegetables

PM Snack: ■ Meal replacement, 1 fruit   *(about 280 calories)*

Dinner: ■ 6 ounces skinless chicken breast, turkey breast, or
(about 500 fish; 1 cup brown rice, whole wheat pasta, or starchy
calories) vegetable; 2 cups steamed vegetables; 1 fruit; salad

---

Total Calories: 1,505   Total Fiber: 30–35 g
Carbs: 222 g—59% cal.   Fat: 18 g—11% cal.   Protein: 113 g—30% cal.

Your Meal Replacement and Portion Control **PROFILE**

Answer the following nine questions to determine how you can achieve your initial weight-loss goals.

DISCOVERING YOUR MEAL PATTERNS

1. Which pattern describes you best?
   ☐ Eat breakfast, lunch, and dinner
   ☐ Skip breakfast, could skip lunch, eat a lot for dinner
   ☐ Diet all the time and skip meals (breakfast or lunch) every day
   ☐ Meals are fine, nighttime snacking is the problem
   ☐ Afternoon snacking followed by a large dinner

CHOOSING YOUR FRUITS AND VEGETABLES

2. List by preference as many of your favorite fruits and vegetables as you can.

MEAL PLANNING

Choose your best option for each meal using the meal plans on pages 72 and 73.

3. Breakfast:
   - ☐ Meal replacement and fruit
   - ☐ Cereal, fat-free milk, and fruit
   - ☐ Egg whites, whole grain bread, and fruit

4. Lunch:
   - ☐ Meal replacement, fruit, and vegetable
   - ☐ Sandwich and fruit/vegetables
   - ☐ Salad with chicken or fish, fruit

5. Snack:
   - ☐ Fruit and rice cake (1,200-calorie plan)
   - ☐ Meal replacement, fruit, and rice cakes (1,500-calorie plan)

6. Dinner:
   - ☐ 3 to 6 ounces (depending on your meal plan) white-meat chicken or turkey, fish, or shellfish
     1 cup rice, pasta, potatoes, or beans
     2 cups steamed vegetables
     Large green salad with no oil dressing, beans, or croutons
     1 fruit

        or

   - ☐ Frozen dinner with less than 300 calories and 25 percent fat
     Large green salad with no oil dressing, beans, or croutons

ESTIMATING YOUR RATE OF WEIGHT LOSS

7. How many calories are you eating now, approximately?

☐ 2,500 ☐ 2,000 ☐ 1,500 ☐ 1,200

8. How many calories will you eat on the meal plan?

☐ 1,500 ☐ 1,200

9. The difference between the calories you eat now and the calories you will eat, divided by 500, equals pounds lost per week; how many pounds will you lose per week?

☐ 1–2 ☐ 2–3 ☐ 3–4

Chapter 5

Educating Your Palate

To this point you have lost some weight, using meal replacements and portion-controlled foods. You have also started to succeed in avoiding the trigger foods and old eating habits that have kept you from losing weight in the past. So what's next?

You are now entering the next and longest-lasting phase of the Resolution Diet. You will learn about how to bring your food intake into balance with those ancient genes that not only hang onto fat and calories, but that also expect you to eat lots of fruits and vegetables. There are two basic sources of food, those based on animal products and those based on plant products. Our bodies have been genetically programmed to handle a diet that is mostly made up of plant foods, such as fruits and vegetables, whole grains, legumes, and tubers. Agriculture and the rise of food processing have led us away from a plant-based diet.

In this chapter, I will introduce you to the California Cuisine Pyramid, a way of eating that is based on the ancient, plant-based diet, and I will tell you how to use vitamins and dietary supplements. Then we will then take a closer look at your food choices, and at ways to make the Resolution Diet work for you.

Finally, I will give you four basic nutritional principles that will guide you to a lifetime of eating without weight gain. To reinforce what you learn, be sure to fill out the profile at the end of the chapter.

Once you educate your palate, you won't be able to eat fatty or overly sweet foods without being put off by them. I know it's hard to believe, but I have experienced it myself and have seen it in my patients. You will want better-tasting foods that are prepared without fat.

A NEW WAY OF EATING: THE CALIFORNIA CUISINE PYRAMID

The pyramid has become a well-recognized teaching tool to encourage changes in eating behavior. At the base, it shows those foods that you should eat the most of each day. At the top, it shows the foods you should eat more selectively.

One of the most commonly used food pyramids comes from the United States Department of Agriculture (USDA). While the USDA pyramid has been a useful aid, it does not go far enough in promoting a plant-based diet. Therefore, my colleagues and I at the UCLA Center for Human Nutrition have developed a new pyramid: the California Cuisine Pyramid. Here are the basic principles on which the California pyramid is based:

- Enjoy nine to eleven servings of vegetables and fruits every day to benefit from their fiber and unique phytonutrients, plant chemicals with health-protecting properties.

- Choose high-fiber breads, cereals, and grains. These healthy choices, along with daily vegetables and fruits, will help meet your need for 25 to 35 grams of fiber per day.

- Consume adequate protein based on your lean body mass, about 0.5 grams of protein per pound of lean body weight. You can meet your protein needs with very-low-fat animal and/or plant foods (see page 84).

- Complement your diet with a daily multivitamin/multimineral supplement, and additional vitamin E, vitamin C, and calcium on the advice of your physician and/or a Registered Dietitian (see page 86).

- Aim for a diet in which you obtain 20 percent of your calories from fat. This provides an amount of fat that most adults can burn off through healthy physical activity while still enjoying their meals.

The Origin of the USDA Food Pyramid

The United States government has been giving advice on how we should eat since 1916, when it issued a food guide for young children. Shortly after that, the government issued a guide based on five food groups. During the 1930s, the government tried to help people shop for food by defining twelve food groups with different cost levels. (One of these, the Thrifty Food Plan, is still used today for the food stamp program.) During World War II, a guide called the Basic Seven was issued.

Then in the mid-1950s, the Basic Four food guide—the one that most people are familiar with—was introduced. By the time I went to medical school in the 1970s, we were taught that you would get all the nutrition you need from these four basic food groups: cereals and grains; fruits and vegetables; milk and dairy products; and meat, beans, and nuts. In 1980, a fifth group was added: fats, oils, and alcohol. The 1980 Hassle-Free Guide also advised people to cut down on fatty meats. This was the first guide to highlight the need to moderate the use of fats, sugars, and alcohol, and to give special attention to calories and dietary fiber.

By 1980, it was evident that more was needed than simple guides that encouraged people to eat more and different types of food. The connection between health and foods was becoming clear. In 1992, after many fits and starts, the Food Guide Pyramid (see page 80, top) was issued. It is a very useful, wide-

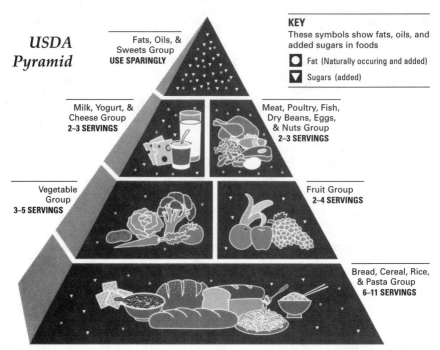

Source: U.S. Department of Agriculture and the U.S. Department of Health and Human Services.

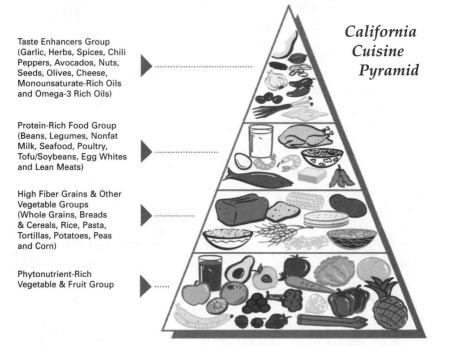

ly recognized tool for teaching the public about different food groups, but it has also been strongly influenced by the food industry. For example, the food-oil producers wanted more triangles and dots, representing fats and sugars, at the top of the pyramid to encourage increased consumption of these foods.

Shifting Focus From the USDA to California Cuisine

The California Cuisine Pyramid (as shown on the previous page, bottom) is a blueprint for our diet in the next century. It differs from the USDA pyramid in several significant ways.

First of all, you will notice that the California Cuisine Pyramid has fruits and vegetables at the bottom, with nine to eleven servings recommended per day, instead of the cereal group shown at the bottom of the USDA pyramid. Besides being relatively low in calories, fruits and vegetables contain phytonutrients that protect against such diseases as cancer and heart disease. Beta-carotene in carrots and lycopene in tomatoes are two examples of these healthful substances. The bulk of your diet should consist of these foods.

The next level of the California pyramid consists of high-fiber cereals and grains. We specify "high-fiber" for a reason. You can eat large portions of low-fiber cereals and pastas because they don't fill you up, with the result that you take in many more calories. The starchy vegetables such as corn and potatoes are on this second level so that these higher-calorie choices won't become the primary way to fulfill the need for a variety of fruits and vegetables each day.

Scientific evidence continues to accumulate that high-fiber foods can help in not only controlling weight, but in preventing disease as well. A recent study, by Dr. David Jacobs at the University of Minnesota School of Public Health, of 35,000 post-menopausal women found that those who ate at least one serving of a whole grain product each day were about 30 percent less likely to die of a heart attack over the nine years of the

study. Whole grains contain fiber, vitamin E, and phytochemi-
cals. These substances are not found in refined grains.

The third level of the pyramid is the protein level. In the USDA
pyramid, it consists of a meat, beans, and nuts group flanked by
a separate dairy group made up of cheese, milk, and yogurt
products. In the California Cuisine Pyramid, there is no separate
dairy group. The benefit of merging the two groups into one protein group from animals or plants is that you will be able to eliminate fat, balance animal and vegetable protein, and meet your
protein requirement each day. However, you must pay extra attention to meeting your daily calcium requirement (see page 87).

The top level contains natural taste enhancers. If you look at
the USDA pyramid you will see that the dots and triangles, representing fats and sugars, sprinkle from the top down through
all the levels of the pyramid. In the California Cuisine Pyramid,
we have spices, nuts, olives, avocados, monounsaturate-rich
oils, and the omega-3 oils found in fish and flaxseed (see page
98) to add taste. Instead of telling consumers to use this level
sparingly, we say "use as needed." Taste is king, and drives the
rest of our pyramid. It is amazing that there are no spices in the
USDA pyramid at all.

So what should you take away from this new pyramid? First
of all, you may have seen the USDA pyramid before, and you
may be puzzled about what constitutes a serving. For the
California pyramid, see "What Is a Serving?" on pages 84 and
85. Second, I believe that 20 percent fat is more than enough to
bring good taste to a diet, while the USDA and most government groups recommend 30 percent. Finally, keep in mind that
pyramids don't tell you everything about a diet. Exercise and
physical activity recommendations are also very important.
Aerobic activities reduce stress and body fat, and weightlifting
boosts lean body mass, increases metabolism, and maintains
healthy bones (see Chapter 7).

An actual menu plan is much more useful than a pyramid, since
you may need less than 1,600 calories to maintain your weight,
even with exercise. (For sample menu plans, see Appendix C.)

All pyramids are based on mythical standard individuals. I don't expect you to take the pyramid literally. I remember that one patient said to me, "You mean I can eat all that, and still lose weight?" The answer is obviously, "No." This is the diet you should be eating when you reach your target weight or when you decide to take a break from losing weight. I would like you to keep the image of your diet as being based on fruits and vegetables. The emphasis is different than current government guidelines in order to emphasize the reduction of fat and sugar and to promote filling foods so that portion control will be easier for you. You will see food pyramids everywhere, from restaurants to cereal boxes. Remember to compare them with the California Cuisine Pyramid in planning your food choices.

Getting Started on a Modified Plant-Based Diet

As you plan your meals, refer to the California Cuisine Pyramid to check that your diet is plant-based. How does this translate into everyday eating? Think of variety. Go beyond the old favorites, such as string beans, peas, and corn, or apples, pears, and oranges. Each fruit and vegetable has its own profile of nutrients and other preventive substances. Dark green leafy and deep orange vegetables provide rich sources of nutrients, and go well together. Try greens, such as collard greens, spinach, kale, and Swiss chard, along with red peppers, sweet pumpkin, carrots, broccoli, and okra. Melons and citrus fruits also have beneficial nutrients. Try papaya, cantaloupe, strawberries, tangerines, kiwi, mango, apricot, and watermelon. Eat legumes, such as pinto, garbanzo, navy, kidney, black, and (no-sugar) baked beans mixed with whole grains, like brown rice, oats, barley, cracked wheat, kasha, couscous, and bulgur. Soybeans and soy foods such as tofu provide a complete protein in many different dishes. Potatoes, sweet potatoes, yams, yucca, taro, turnip, and jicama are in the root and tuber category of plants.

What Is a Serving?

Food Group	Serving Size	How Many a Day?*	
		1,600 cal/day	2,200 cal/day
Fruits and vegetables	1 cup raw leafy vegetables	5	7
	1/2 cup chopped raw or cooked vegetables		
	1 medium fresh fruit	4	4
	1 cup berries or melon		
High-fiber grains and other vegetables	1 slice whole grain bread	6	10
	1/2 cup cooked whole grain cereal, whole wheat pasta, or brown rice		
	1 oz. (28 g) whole grain cold cereal		
	1/2 cup potatoes, peas, or corn		
Protein-rich foods	3 oz. cooked skinless chicken breast (27 g)	50 to 60	70 to 80
	3 oz. cooked skinless turkey breast (25 g)		
	3 oz. cooked seafood (16–22 g)		
	1/2 cup tofu or tempeh (10–20 g)		
	1/2 cup beans or legumes (7–9 g)		
	1 cup nonfat milk or plain yogurt (8 g)		
	3 egg whites (11 g)		

What Is a Serving?

Food Group	Serving Size	How Many a Day?*	
		1,600 cal/day	2,200 cal/day
Taste enhancers	Garlic, herbs, spices, chili peppers, dried fruit, jams, avocados, nuts, seeds, olives, cheese, monounsaturate-rich oils (olive, canola), and omega 3-rich oils (fish, flaxseed)	below 200 cal	below 300 cal

* The pyramid's suggested range of servings provides approximately 1,600 to 2,200 calories per day of low-fat, high-fiber food choices. Your individual calorie needs may be higher or lower based on your age, sex, weight, and level of physical activity. Consult a knowledgeable physician and/or Registered Dietitian to tailor the pyramid to your unique needs.

There is room for meat in the modified plant-based diet. The secret is to not let meat dominate the meal. As you use meats in your diet, think of them in the same way you think of ketchup or mustard—as a source of increased taste. Instead of a big hamburger with some ketchup and mustard, think of the vegetables as the center for your sandwich—eggplant, zucchini, peppers, onions, and carrot strips—plus a thin slice or two of chicken or turkey. A general rule is that meat should not occupy more than a third of your plate. Also, stay away from "mock" meats, such as mock steak made with almonds and oil. The idea is to not base your diet on the taste and texture of meat.

Dairy products are a rich source of calcium and certain other minerals, along with vitamins and protein. They should be consumed only in nonfat form to minimize extra calories. Two glasses of whole milk provide over 600 mg of calcium, but they also have a lot of calories (see page 87). So don't change your whole diet just based on calcium intake, since you can take calcium supplements. You still will want to balance animal and plant protein, and milk products count as animal protein.

Beyond these choices are thousands of exotic fruits and vegetables. There are over 150,000 edible plant species on earth, and we eat only a small number of them. Increasing the diversity of your vegetables and fruits means that you will be getting more nutrients for better health. Think of exploring this interesting collection of international foods as an adventure on which you are about to embark. Eating a wide variety of plant-based foods is a good way to ensure that you never regain weight (as long as you do not go back to eating your trigger foods) ever again.

SUPPLEMENTS THAT COMPLETE A HEALTHY DIET

As you have learned throughout this book, our food supply is not designed to be healthy, just profitable. It would be wonderful if you could get all the nutrition you need from eating the four basic food groups, but it is simply not possible. Most Americans don't eat regularly from enough different foods. While you could get 500 milligrams of vitamin C from eating fruits and vegetables, most of us don't. You would have to eat about 5,000 calories a day to get 400 International Units (IU) of vitamin E in your food. Folic acid, which has been shown to be so important for preventing birth defects, heart disease, and possibly cancer, is found in dark green, leafy lettuces such as collard greens. The richest sources in our diets are fortified breakfast cereals, and these don't usually have enough to be protective.

As a parallel to the basic four food groups, I like to recommend the basic four supplements. These are a multivitamin/multimineral pill and three additional supplements: 400 IU of vitamin E, 500 milligrams of vitamin C, and 500 or 1,000 milligrams of calcium, depending on how much you are getting from your diet. (To learn why I recommend calcium supplements over dairy products, see "At What Cost Calcium?" on the next page.) Women need a total of 1,000 milligrams of calcium per day before age fifty and 1,500 milligrams per day after

At What Cost Calcium?

Dairy products are often recommended as a good calcium source. They are, but at a high calorie cost. To eat enough dairy products to get 1,000 milligrams of calcium a day, you would have to eat the following amounts of various dairy foods.

Dairy Product	Calories	Fat (grams)
5 1-oz. slices cheddar cheese	570	47
6 1-oz. slices American cheese	560	42
4 1-oz. slices Swiss cheese	428	31
3 8-oz. glasses whole milk	450	31
3 8-oz. glasses reduced-fat milk (2%)	360	15
3 8-oz. glasses skim milk (fat-free)	240	1.2

By choosing skim, or fat-free, milk, you can get your calcium with a minimum of extra calories and fat. You can better use those calories elsewhere.

age fifty. Men need 800 to 1,000 milligrams per day. I put these vitamins out on my breakfast table. You may want to do this at dinner instead. In either case, I advise taking vitamins with food, since they are always better absorbed with a meal.

A CLOSER LOOK AT YOUR FOOD CHOICES

As you continue to strengthen your resolution and change your diet, you will find yourself beginning to read food labels. This is an important part of your palate's education. You will learn how to avoid the hidden fats and sweets in the foods you buy. You will also learn how to find the best-quality protein.

Eliminating Hidden Fats and Sweets

As you read labels, you will begin to notice the hidden fat in many food categories. You should know how many calories you are getting each time you indulge in trigger foods and related treats. I believe you will find that you are better off

Substitution Strategies for Specific Foods

You might be surprised at just how big a difference some simple food substitutions can make in terms of calories and fat. Here are some examples.

Example 1: *Nuts vs. Popcorn*

1 cup of peanuts, dry roasted	*814 calories*	*70.5 grams of fat*
6 tablespoons of peanut butter	*564 calories*	*48 grams of fat*
vs.		
3 cups of air-popped popcorn	*45 calories*	*0.5 grams of fat*

You save: *500 to 800 calories and 50 to 70 grams of fat*

Example 2: *Red Meat vs. Chicken Breast*

9 ounces lean sirloin steak	*987 calories*	*43 grams of fat*
9 ounces lean pork chop	*570 calories*	*39 grams of fat*
vs.		
3 ounces chicken breast	*147 calories*	*4 grams of fat*

You save: *400 to 800 calories and 35 to 40 grams of fat*

Example 3: *Whole Milk vs. Skim (Fat-Free) Milk*

8 ounces whole milk	*150 calories*	*8 grams of fat*
vs.		
8 ounces skim (fat-free) milk	*86 calories*	*trace of fat*

You save: *64 calories and 8 grams of fat*

Example 4: *Eliminating 2 Ounces of Cheese From a Sandwich*

2 ounces American processed cheese	*212 calories*	*18 grams of fat*

You save: *212 calories and 18 grams of fat*

without the trigger foods most of the time. There is no way to have your cake without the calories that go with it, but at least you will know what degree of compromise you are making each time.

I believe that it is better to know that you are eating something you should not be eating, rather than think that you can simply make so-called low-fat choices. As you persist in making the right choices, you will lose the cravings that control your eating habits. I hope that in the future, gourmet chefs will use only the fat and natural sweeteners in foods themselves. A

Example 5: *Having Wine or Beer Instead of a Pina Colada*

4.5 ounces pina colada mixed drink   346 calories
vs.
12 ounces light beer 100 calories or 4 ounces light wine   80 calories
You save: *250 to 300 calories*

Example 6: *French Fries or Onion Rings vs. Steamed Vegetables*

20 French fried potatoes	*316 calories*	*16 grams of fat*
7 fried onion rings	*285 calories*	*19 grams of fat*
vs.		
½ cup squash-zucchini, steamed	*14 calories*	*0.1 grams of fat*
½ cup broccoli, steamed	*23 calories*	*0.2 grams of fat*

You save: *260 to 300 calories and 16 to 19 grams of fat*

Example 7: *Green Tossed Salad with Grilled Chicken Breast and Balsamic Vinegar vs. a Large Chinese Chicken Salad*

Chinese chicken salad	*1,014 calories*	*61 grams of fat*
vs.		
Green tossed salad	*210 calories*	*4 grams of fat*

You save: *800 calories and 57 grams of fat*

Altogether, these changes save up to 3,300 calories. This is about 1 pound of fat. Imagine how many calories you could save each day by making wise choices and educating your palate to avoid fats and sweets. As you read labels, play this game and you will see that you are saving up to 1,000 calories per day by simply making the right choices.

---

slice of creamy avocado or nonfat cheese can do a lot for the experience of eating. Tasty natural recipes can be found in magazines and books (see Appendix A), but every day you will find hidden fat/sweet traps out there—see "Substitution Strategies for Specific Foods" above.

The latest diet idea has been that you should get adequate protein. Unfortunately, the emphasis on protein has also resulted in less attention being paid to carbohydrates, including sugars. When you are losing weight, you are burning fat calories from your body that you have removed from your diet. The balance of your diet should be protein and carbohydrates, with as little fat as necessary to make your food taste good. Excess sugar as well as fat represent additional calories you just don't need. When you read labels, look for these other names for sugar: honey, dates, orange juice, maltodextrin, and corn sugars. The government allows sugars added as chains of five or more sugar molecules to be listed not as sugars but as "complex" carbohydrates. In fact, these corn-sugar derivatives act just like sugar after they dissolve in your stomach.

Artificial sweeteners are another bugaboo. I often see an overweight woman adding some artificial sweetener to her coffee to save a few calories and then turn right around and eat a piece of cheesecake. This is not an accident. The artificial sweeteners are sweeter than sugar and make you crave sweet desserts; avoid them. Read the label and you will find the first ingredient is sugar (nonnutritive dextrose), the second is sand (calcium silicate), and the third is a tiny amount of the oversweet chemical sweetener.

One easy place to find extra sugar in your diet is in nonfat or fat-free yogurt. An eight-ounce cup of low-fat yogurt with fruit on the bottom can have 6 teaspoons of added sugar; a glass of chocolate fat-free milk has 4. That's up to 240 calories in a snack (not a meal) that you can finish in minutes. Let me give you some examples (in the list below) of differences in calories and why it is important to read labels if you are including plain nonfat yogurt in a meal.

Calorie Content of Yogurt

Yogurt	Serving Size	Calories
Fat-free, plain	8 oz.	110
Low-fat, fruit on the bottom	8 oz.	240
Fat-free with fruit	8 oz.	200
Caramel/chocolate topped	6 oz.	210
Fat-free chunky fruit	6 oz.	160
Fat- and sugar-free	4.4 oz.	70

As the calories go down, so does the amount of beneficial calcium. The serving of 70-calorie yogurt has only 10 percent of the daily calcium requirement, compared with 40 percent in the serving of 110-calorie yogurt. So for only an extra 40 calories, you get much more calcium. These are important trade-offs that affect the quality of your whole diet.

Eating the Right Amount of the Best Proteins

Protein is also listed on food labels, and now that you have sugars, fats, and calories under control, let's look at protein. Your exact protein requirement depends on how much lean body mass you have (if you haven't done so already, see Chapter 2 to learn how to determine your lean body mass). You need to eat 0.5 grams of protein per day for every pound of lean tissue.

The best-quality proteins give you the most easily assimilated proteins per calorie of food. These include egg whites, milk protein, and soy protein. They have an ideal mixture of the amino-acid protein building blocks that our bodies expect. Meats and fish are about 80 percent as good in terms of amino-acid content. Beans, corn, and rice are each individually between 20 and 40 percent as good as the best proteins, but when you combine beans or other legumes (such as lentils) with rice, corn, or wheat, you get a protein that is as good as more-expensive meats. That is why strict vegetarians combine these types of proteins, and more vegetarians are eating soy protein as protein powders, tofu, and soy burgers. Even if you are not a vegetarian, eating more plant-based protein is not a bad idea.

What does 0.5 gram per pound of lean mass really mean? Let's make it simple. Three ounces of meat is about the size of the palm of your hand. Have this much at lunch and dinner if you are of average build. If you have a larger build, eat two palmfuls, or 6 ounces, at dinner. For breakfast have a meal replacement shake, or if you have some milk on your cereal, be sure to have a full glass in total. If you are having eggs, eat two or three hard-boiled or poached eggs with as little yellow as possible.

Following these simple rules will allow you to balance your protein and carbohydrates easily without carrying around a calculator to figure protein and carbohydrate exchanges. Your body has ways to adjust to your diet, so don't sweat the small stuff.

THE RESOLUTION DIET AND THE EDUCATED PALATE

I know that adopting the modified plant-based diet shown in the California Cuisine Pyramid may take a bit of an adjustment on your part. That's OK—you don't have to worry about being perfect. Don't fret if you don't make the correct food choices every time. By taking a tailored, individualized approach, you can work on those issues that most apply to you. This will allow you to control your weight for as long as you live.

Tolerating Some Trigger Foods

There is clearly an advantage in going "cold turkey" on your particular trigger foods. If I advise someone to stop smoking, I don't tell them to smoke filtered cigarettes. Similarly, if cheese is a problem for you, I am not going to advise you to eat nonfat cheese. If red meat is a problem for you, then I will not suggest that you look for low-fat cuts of meat. Instead, I will tell you to put steak sauce on white meat of chicken or turkey and pretend it's red meat.

I picked the trigger foods listed in Chapter 3 for both behavioral and nutrition reasons, but there are individual exceptions. If there is nonfat cheese (or sour cream, or fat-free whip or mayo) in a dish, and you know what the total calories are, go for it. Nonfat cheese is a good source of protein, but that doesn't warrant eating four slices, with their 320 calories, right out of the fridge. Similarly, if there is a walnut in your salad, go ahead and eat it just this time. Just don't eat a bag of nuts as a snack. The idea is to not feel deprived while not eating enough of the trigger foods to go back to your old, uncontrolled habits. The key is to stop eating trigger foods unless you have them in a recipe, so you know that the total calories and fat content have been controlled.

Changing Your Taste Buds

Your taste buds are the first parts of your body to encounter food, but taste originates with your sense of smell. For example, people who lose their sense of smell complain that their foods don't taste the same. The visual appearance of foods also contributes to the desire to eat, since it can trigger the release of certain hormones into your bloodstream that make you feel hungry. These inputs from vision, smell, and taste are all put together in a center in your brain called the hypothalamus. All of the functions controlled in this center are critical to life, and retaining fat is no exception (to learn why, see page 16).

It is possible to change your taste buds, which respond to the environment just as other parts of your body do. For example, if you sit in a darkened room, your eyes will adapt to the dark in a few minutes, and you will then be able to see. Your tongue senses four basic tastes: sweet, sour, salty, and bitter. The tongue also responds to the taste enhancer glutamate, an amino acid that is added to many processed foods (and which gives some people headaches).

Beyond these basic tastes, fat is a taste enhancer. There is no daily requirement for fat, because in our society it is impossible to not get the fat calories you need. On the other hand, you can easily get hooked on excess fat, since it increases the other tastes of foods. In ancient times, humans found themselves in a calorie-poor environment, so a craving for fat made sense. Despite this inborn tendency, you can change your taste buds. But you will have to be willing to make some real changes in the types of foods you eat. (For some help in this area, see "How to Recognize and Control Food Cravings" on page 94.) By cutting fat and refined sugar, eating reasonable portions, and increasing (through exercise) the rate at which you burn calories, you give your brain a chance to regulate your weight.

How to Recognize and Control Food Cravings

Food cravings are often not driven by hunger, and they do not activate the normal triggering centers in the brain that lead to a feeling of fullness. I will explain a few of the common food cravings that I have encountered. There are two general approaches to cravings. First, you can confront the craving by realizing what you are doing and talking yourself out of it. When you succeed, congratulate yourself. Second, you can displace the craving by doing something else. The more active you can be in distracting yourself, the better.

If You Have a Sweet Tooth

If you crave sweets, the first step is to avoid artificial sweeteners. These little packets are sweeter than sugar and will simply cause your sweet tooth to get worse. Instead, substitute freshly cut fruits for ice cream or cake at dessert. Learn to turn down hot fudge sundaes by using (silent) self-congratulation for doing so. You can have a sweet meal replacement, such as Ultra Slim-Fast, frozen with coffee crystals or sliced bananas. When eaten with fruit, this can be a filling meal with a rich taste. You can also make a fresh fruit sorbet in a blender using ice and your favorite fruit.

If You Have Cheese Cravings

If you crave cheese, don't turn to nonfat cheeses. By having something that looks like cheese, you are maintaining the cheese habit. Instead, wean yourself off cheese. If you don't buy it, you won't eat it. I am more interested in what you eat every day than I am in having you completely off of cheese for the rest of your life. I tell my patients to go ahead and have a great slice of fatty Swiss cheese with a fine glass of red wine while on vacation. I simply don't want you eating "cheese food," whether or not it is "nonfat," on an everyday basis. Soon your taste buds will no longer crave cheese.

Variety, Spice, and Satiety

How do you cut your portion sizes? One of the best ways is to increase the variety and taste of your foods. Spicy and tasty foods are more likely to satisfy your appetite than bland, sweet, creamy foods. In general, these more varied foods will have more nutrients, including vitamins and minerals, than higher-fat foods. Try using ginger, scallions, onions, and garlic in your cooking. Chili peppers are another wonderful way to increase

---

If You Have Trouble Feeling Full

Have you ever had trouble feeling full after a healthy meal? This type of hunger can be controlled. Learn to use fiber and water before you sit down to eat. You can buy a fiber product made with psyllium seed in either powder (such as psyllium seed husks or Metamucil) or tablet form. Have some water with the fiber (never take it dry) before you eat, and you will have an easier time in controlling portion sizes. You should also use a plate with subdivided sections similar to those used in frozen dinners, and only bring the specific portions to the table. Don't finish other people's portions, and don't eat leftover foods as you clean up after dinner. Finally, once dinner is finished, leave the kitchen. If you have to, place no-binge reminders on the refrigerator. If you can't stop yourself, use air-popped popcorn as a temporary crutch. At least you will be getting fewer calories per bite.

If You Like It Sweet, Fat, and Creamy

Ice cream, cream pies, whipped cream, and flavored yogurts provide the combination of sweet, fatty, and creamy tastes that some dieters crave. This is an acquired craving that will disappear once you stop eating the foods that stimulate this craving. I don't recommend using the imitation, so-called nonfat whipped creams, since they will only maintain your craving. Instead, stick with frozen meal replacements and whip them up in a blender. The taste won't be quite as creamy, and so your taste buds will shift. Soon you will find that you no longer crave sweet, creamy desserts.

Conquering any of these behavior patterns can require a concentrated effort over a period of time. Do not expect these habits to go away suddenly. Eventually, you will be successful.

---

eating satisfaction. It has been shown that eating hot chilis can result in the release of endorphins, the hormones in the brain that cause pleasurable sensations. Chili peppers also raise body temperature. In one study, chilis were shown to cause a small amount of weight loss when added to the diet. The authors of this study speculated that the increase in body temperature burned off the fat.

No matter how they work, I believe that spices can help you

be satisfied with smaller volumes of food. Many different ethnic cuisines use particular spices. Here's a brief list of the spices that can be used to prepare various ethnic dishes without a lot of added fat:

- Asian: garlic, scallion, onion, ginger, low-sodium soy sauce
- Mediterranean: oregano, basil, tomato, garlic, scallions
- Mexican and Latin American: cilantro, tomato, green and red chili peppers, onion
- Cajun: chili peppers, cajun chili sauces, blackening spice mix

Look at cookbooks from these various ethnic cuisines, and at some of the newer fusion cuisines that combine two or more culinary traditions. This will help you get beyond ketchup and yellow mustard to some great new tastes.

Focus on Your Eating Habits

Eating should be the focus of your activities at the table so that you can really taste your food. Do not read the paper or watch television while eating. You should eat on a regularly scheduled basis, so that you are not famished when you first sit down to eat. Eat slowly, and put your fork down between bites. As you eat, focus on the tastes of the food you are eating. These steps will help your normal hunger-control mechanisms work as they should. As you eat, try to distinguish true hunger from food cravings. You should be eating in response to hunger and stopping when you are no longer hungry. If you are eating out of control, you are probably being driven by cravings.

THE FOUR BASIC NUTRITION PRINCIPLES

Principles are rules that you can live by. Steven Covey, in *Seven Habits of Highly Effective People,* talks a lot about principle-centered living. Here are my four basic nutrition principles that you will be using in the Resolution Diet.

Eat Only the Fat You Can Burn, and Eat the Right Kinds of Fat

Remember, the most important hidden source of extra calories is fat. You can get perfectly good taste by eating a diet that consists of 20 percent fat, instead of the 30-percent fat diet recommended by the USDA and others, and not have those extra calories to burn. It is no longer true that you have to use lots of added fat to make foods taste good.

There are fats that are essential to health, though, and you must include them in your diet. You need about 5 to 10 percent of your total calories from fat to consist of two particular fatty acids: linoleic and linolenic acids. These are called the essential fatty acids, and they come in two basic types, omega-3 acids (linolenic) and omega-6 acids (linoleic). They are needed by the body for everything from cholesterol regulation to proper immune function. Vegetables such as corn naturally contain these fats, together with natural vitamin E.

The problem is that the omega-3s and omega-6s have gotten out of balance in the modern diet. The oil manufacturers have stripped the linolenic acid out of corn oil, since it reduces the oil's shelf life. In the process, much of the vitamin E is also removed. This leaves you with an excess intake of linoleic acid, which is converted to arachidonic acid. Arachidonic acid promotes the production of other signals in your body that in turn promote heart disease and cancer.

At one time, all of the so-called polyunsaturated fats were thought to be good for you by comparison with the saturated fats from red meats. In fact, increased intake of corn oil and other polyunsaturated fats (including safflower, soybean, and cottonseed oils) promotes weight gain, which in turn can cause higher cholesterol levels. There are no calorie-free "good" fats; all fats have 140 calories per tablespoon. But there is an advantage to ensuring that the fat you do eat comes from either fish or plant sources of monounsaturated and omega-3-rich oils. Monounsaturated fatty acids are found in olive oil, avocados, nuts, and seeds. Omega-3 fatty acids are found in fish in the forms of eicosapentaenoic acid (EPA) and docosahexaenoic acid (DHA). Fish has less saturated fat than red meat or chicken, as long as you buy it fresh and cook it at home without creamy, fatty sauces. (Fish at restaurants can be full of added fat you don't know about.) Total fat and the amount of omega-3 fat in different types of fish vary greatly (see below).

Omega-3 Content of Fish

Fish (6 oz. cooked)	Total Fat (g)	Omega-3 Fat (g)
Atlantic salmon, farmed	21	3.7
Atlantic salmon, wild	14	3.1
Fish sticks (6)	21	0.4
Catfish, farmed	14	0.3
Coho salmon, farmed	14	2.2
Coho salmon, wild	7	1.8
Rainbow trout, farmed	12	2.0
Rainbow trout, wild	10	1.7
Swordfish	9	1.4

Plant foods such as flaxseed and purslane contain alpha linolenic acid (ALA), a fatty acid similar to DHA and EPA. The body can make DHA and EPA from ALA, but it is not clear that it acts exactly like fish oils in the body.

The natural omega-3 fatty acids found in low-fat fish are beneficial, and eating fish as a major protein source in addition to chicken, turkey, and soy can be helpful in balancing your fats. As we saw in Chapter 4, you should avoid high-fat fish when you are trying to lose weight. But when you are maintaining your weight, you can eat fish that is rich in omega-3s, as listed above. Just be careful to not forget about calories altogether. Your body will adjust and balance the mix of fats you eat, as long as you unload the great excess of hidden fats from vegetable oils in your diet.

Don't Simply Replace Fat With Sugar

Recently, there has been an epidemic increase in obesity in this country, from 24 to 32 percent of the population. This was at a time when there were more than 1,000 fat-free foods on the market. How could this happen? Reduced physical activity, high stress levels, and sweet treats resulted in more fat being deposited than burned. As we saw in Chapter 3, the body can convert sugar to fat very efficiently, but the word "fat-free" sells food. Pretzels, which were always fat-free, are labeled as fat-free to draw attention to themselves. Fat-free yogurts with lots of added sugar are sold as snack treats providing lots of extra calories. I once had a patient who gained 30 pounds eating three servings a day of low-fat yogurt in addition to her regular meals.

As I've said before, sugar is not evil. If total calories are controlled, sugar is a nutrient your body likes to use. In fact, it will convert extra protein into sugars before depositing them as fat, and it can even convert some fat to sugar. But you cannot cut all the fat from a typical American high-fat diet, replace it with sugar, and expect to lose weight. As far as your body is concerned, fat and sugar are both ways of saying "calorie."

Lose the Fat, But Keep the Muscle

Many dieters, in a rush to lose weight, quickly stop eating. During the first few weeks of starvation, 50 percent of the weight you lose is from your lean muscle tissue. Yo-yo dieters, who go on and off diets, progressively lose more and more muscle. This has several bad consequences. First, it lowers the number of calories you burn each day (remember, muscle tissue burns more calories than does fat), making you likely to regain the weight. Second, it makes you weaker, and weakens your bones. Many women who skip protein at breakfast and lunch—bagel and coffee for breakfast, meatless salad for lunch—lose 15 to 20 pounds of lean tissue when they diet. This lowers the number of at-rest calories they burn each day by up to 300 calories per day.

If you have done this, don't worry. I will tell you how to rebuild your muscle in Chapter 7, but for now it is important to remember that you must eat an adequate amount of protein. You will find it very easy to meet your daily protein requirement by adding a little protein to each meal. It's not as big a deal as some diet plans would have you think. There is no evidence that lots of extra protein is important unless you are a serious weightlifter building extra muscle. If you eat extra protein and fail to incorporate it into muscle, your body will simply make fat from it. By the way, the popular notion that excess protein is somehow associated with kidney disease has never been proven. Actually, a considerable percentage of patients with kidney disease have the type of diabetes that is strongly associated with obesity, and which is promoted by a high-fat diet.

My colleagues and I are doing research involving middle-aged men to see if increasing the protein requirement from 0.5 grams per pound of lean mass to 0.8 grams per pound makes a difference when they are building muscle through an aggressive exercise program. But right now, if you just stick with the protein requirement discussed on page 91, you'll be fine.

Fill Up With Fiber

Fiber, while it doesn't provide nutrients or calories, does serve an important health function in moving foods through the digestive tract. Modern breakfast cereals were first produced in the nineteenth century by Dr. Kellogg, a physician who believed that cereals would detoxify the human body. (I often think of Kellogg as the Nathan Pritikin of his time.) Although he didn't know exactly how cereals cleansed the body, Kellogg was right. We now know that the fiber in whole grains absorbs hormones, bile acids, drugs, and some toxins in the intestines and carries them out of the body.

It is still true today that a high-fiber cereal can help you reach the goal of eating 25 to 35 daily grams of fiber, the amount recommended by the National Cancer Institute to help prevent colon cancer. You can also get fiber from the fruits and vegetables I have recommended in Chapter 3, which is why I listed their fiber contents. A good meal replacement has 5 grams of fiber per serving. Fiber supplements can also be used to reach the 25- to 35-gram goal.

That great philosopher of modern civilization, Mel Brooks, once said, "Beans, beans, the musical fruit, the more you eat the more you toot!" In fact, your body will adjust to the gas-producing effects of fiber over a few weeks, and you will be much healthier from then on. If you have an irritable bowel or spastic colon already, see your doctor before adding lots of fiber. I use fiber in treating many of my patients, but this is an individual matter for you and your physician to decide.

The California Cuisine Pyramid provides you with a plan that is easy to use and will make it easier for you to maintain your weight. Lower-fat, higher-fiber choices lead to more filling with less calories and more nutrition. If you have had an easy time losing weight, you will probably maintain your weight using this approach. On the other hand, if you have a very slow metabolism, this approach will have to be coupled with exercise and portion control to maintain your weight. If you regain, you can always go back to Chapter 4 for a refresher course. The strategies you will learn in the next chapter will help you keep the promise of permanent weight loss every day.

Your Personal Palate-Education Plan
PROFILE

Answer the following fourteen questions to determine how you can achieve your palate-education goals.

FOLLOWING THE CALIFORNIA CUISINE PYRAMID

1. Reread the list of fruits and vegetables that you compiled in the Chapter 4 profile. Are there any new fruits and vegetables that you would like to try?

2. How could you increase your fiber intake to reach 25 to 35 grams per day?

3. Are you getting protein at each meal? List your proteins in a typical day.

4. Which are your favorite spices? (check all that apply)

☐ Chili   ☐ Onion   ☐ Mustard

☐ Garlic   ☐ Ginger   ☐ Ketchup

☐ Scallions

GETTING YOUR SUPPLEMENTS

5. Do you take supplements now?

☐ Yes   ☐ No

6. If yes, what supplements do you take?

WAYS OF SAVING FAT AND CALORIES

7. Check any of the following calorie-saving ideas that you plan to try:

☐ Popcorn vs. nuts

☐ Chicken vs. red meat

☐ Cheese elimination

☐ Wine or light beer vs. cocktails and liquor

☐ Steamed vegetables vs. French fries or onion rings

☐ Fat-free (skim) milk vs. whole milk

8. Can you find two ways to save calories on your own by label reading? (See page 42.)

FOCUSING ON YOUR CRAVINGS

9. Circle the rating that applies to you for each craving; rate
each from 1 to 5, with 1 being no craving at all.

Sweet tooth	1	2	3	4	5
Cheese craving	1	2	3	4	5
Stomach stuffing	1	2	3	4	5
Sweet, fat, creamy	1	2	3	4	5

10. Do you have a problem with portion control?

☐ Yes   ☐ No

11. If yes, how can you combat it?

12. Can you think of self-talk for confronting your cravings?

13. Can you think of two ways of diverting your cravings?

FOCUSING ON YOUR EATING HABITS

14. What are your eating habits?
☐ Do you watch TV or read while eating?
☐ Do you pause while eating?
☐ Do you leave some food on the plate?

Chapter 6

Living the Resolution Diet

A t this point you have all of the key principles you need to make your Resolution Diet a success. But living your resolution in the real world is not always easy. I think most diets fail because while they sound great in theory, they don't account for the way you actually live your life. A diet plan cannot account for a crying baby, unpaid bills, or a demanding boss. That's why I now want to give you some very practical strategies that can help you to overcome everyday challenges to your resolution, challenges that can throw you off your plan unless you are prepared.

The first step in taking control of your diet is to separate eating from those times and activities that stimulate uncontrolled eating. As with the Trigger Food Strategy, what we are talking about now is a trigger situation strategy. Every day you will plan for the high-risk situations, identify them whenever they happen, change your behavior, and, most importantly, recognize your success and pat yourself on the back. Also, learn from your mistakes and try not to repeat them.

In this chapter, I will share with you many of the hints I have picked up, both from my own experiences in struggling with the problem of maintaining a healthy diet and from talking to thousands of patients over the years. They cover eating at home and at work, and eating in a variety of social situations, including going to restaurants. The goal is to be able to follow your Resolution Diet every day and everywhere you find yourself. Use this chapter's profile to keep track of your particular problem areas.

HOW TO EAT AT HOME

While eating at home has become less common, as we all run about in our fast-paced lives, home is still the place where you begin to keep your resolution. That's true no matter how many meals a day you eat there.

Overall Strategies for Eating at Home

Living your resolution starts in the kitchen, where you store the supplies that permit you to binge on the wrong foods.

❑ *Identify the problem foods.* Let's look at a typical high-risk situation at home. You are about to sit down to watch a football game or your favorite situation comedy. You go to the kitchen to get your favorite snack. You eat rapidly without tasting the snack, and go back to the kitchen. Now you pick up some leftovers from the refrigerator. By the time the TV show or game is over, you feel both full and guilty.

Now let's go back and use our trigger situation strategy.

If it's not in your pantry, you can't eat it. So let's start by cleaning out the junk from your favorite kitchen cabinet. You know the one! It's where you look when the commercial comes on, or when you get bored or antsy at night. Go ahead. Get rid of the chocolate chip cookies and the potato chips. Replace them with popcorn kernels, so that you can make some air-popped popcorn. Take a good look at the refrigerator. Take your leftovers and toss or freeze them, so that they won't be available for evening gorging. Toss that fat-free ice cream. You will be having a frozen meal replacement instead. Open the butter compartment. Throw out the fat-free margarine. Can't believe it's not butter? I can't either—throw it out! Mayonnaise has to go. Can't bear to throw food away? Give unopened food to a food bank, or give your goodies to a neighbor or relative.

❑ *Create a safe zone.* Once you clean out the kitchen, it's time to restock with fresh, nonfattening foods. I strongly urge you to find a good source of fruits and vegetables, especially if your local supermarket's produce section isn't all it should be. Find another supermarket, or look for a store that specializes in produce. See if your neighborhood has a farmer's market, where you can buy fresh, locally grown produce.

Once the pantry and refrigerator are in shape, don't forget the spice rack. A rack full of dusty, grimy bottles is not going to make you want to substitute spiciness for fattiness or sweetness in your cooking. If you can't remember the last time you used a spice, throw it out. Buy only the spices you like and will use often, so that they remain fresh and flavorful.

Breakfast Strategies

There are several ways you can make eating breakfast at home a low-calorie experience.

❑ *Make sure you eat breakfast.* If you are not in the habit of eating breakfast every day, start developing that habit now. Eating breakfast keeps you from getting too hungry later on, and gives you the nourishment you need to get through the morning. It also adds some balance to your daily meal planning.

Once you decide to make breakfast a daily feature, you must make healthy breakfast choices based on your lifestyle and weight-loss goals:

• Even if you hate eating in the mornings, you can always have a basic breakfast, including a meal replacement, a fruit, and a cup of coffee. It is convenient, easy, and inexpensive. You can plan your breakfast when you travel by taking along some ready-to-drink meal replacements. Skipping breakfast or just having coffee and a bagel is not a good idea. This will give you carbohydrates and no protein. As a result, you will be hungry again in a few hours.

• You can have a more complete breakfast when you have more time, but are still rushing out the door. You should select a high-fiber cereal, such as All-Bran or 40% Bran Flakes. Limit the serving to 1 cup with 8 ounces of nonfat milk, which provides the protein. A small banana or a fruit plate of cantaloupe, honeydew melon, and a few strawberries rounds out this breakfast. Avoid fruit juices, especially orange juice, which is pure sugar and can provide 160 calories in a small glass. Instead, eat a whole orange or half of a grapefruit. By the way, throw away your grapefruit spoon with the serrated edges. Peal the grapefruit and eat it as you would an orange. That way you will be getting the fibrous white coating inside the grapefruit, which contains healthy, filling dietary fibers.

• On weekends, you can have what I call the Sunday breakfast. You have more time to enjoy breakfast, which means you can consider other sources of protein. Poach or boil two or three eggs, using as little yellow as possible or no yolk at all. In addition, have some fruit, a slice of high-fiber wheat bread, and a cup of coffee. If you are still hungry, have a small bowl of high-fiber cereal with nonfat milk. But that's it.

❏ *Know when breakfast is over.* You must start your day. Don't linger at the breakfast table—it's easy to do if you do not have a job that takes you out of the house. Don't eat the food left behind by other members of the family. Get your day going and have some plans that take you out of the house in the morning. Go for a walk after breakfast. Just do something so that you get out of the kitchen.

Lunch Strategies

Lunch at home is a snap with these simple strategies.

❑ *Plan your lunches.* Lunch is easy. If you want to have a meal replacement and a fruit, decide in advance how many days you would like to do this each week, up to five days a week if you wish. Have your meal replacement ready to go in the refrigerator. Another good lunch is half of a sandwich with 3 ounces of tuna, turkey, or chicken, and a fruit such as an apple. If that is not enough for you, have some cut-up vegetables, such as carrots or celery. If you like salads, you can cut up the tuna, turkey, or chicken on top of the salad. With lunch have water or unsweetened iced tea.

❑ *Know when lunch is over.* Have something to do after lunch. Chores that take you out of the house are a good way to avoid overeating if you are at home. If you plan to be away from the house at lunch, you can take your meal replacement or bagged sandwich with you.

I know that sometimes it is difficult to get out of the house if you have young children. Are there other parents on your block that you can get together with? (Tell them about what you're doing, and maybe you can all go on the Resolution Diet together.) Often, parents who don't live on the same block will form play groups and take their children to each others' houses. (Politely turn down any cake or cookies you may be offered.) Or you can hire a baby sitter for one or two afternoons a week. And don't forget the local library, which may have story hours and other activities for you and your children to enjoy together.

Dinner Strategies

Even in today's fast-paced world, a homecooked dinner can enrich family life. Use the strategies below to make dinner a low-fat feast.

❏ *Plan your meals.* No matter whether you are a naturally great cook or you can't boil water, it is possible to combine healthy ingredients into a great meal. By simply changing the way you shop and cook in little ways, you will be able to provide yourself and your family with a low-fat diet. The best way to do this is to use a weekly meal plan (see Appendix C for some to get you started), and base your shopping list on the plan. Remember, no extras!

❏ *Use low-fat/no-fat ingredients.* Your meals will be as healthy as the ingredients you use in them. Stay away from oil-based cooking, such as sautéing, and stick with steaming, broiling, or baking. If you must use oil, stick with olive oil, and use the smallest amount possible. Even better, use a *lightly* applied olive oil-based cooking spray. Stay away from high-fat extras, such as cheese, butter, mayonnaise, and dressing. For ideas on how to use specific ingredients, see "Low-Fat Cooking for Different Foods" on the next page.

❏ *Use frozen dinners for portion control.* Your evening meal can be a frozen portion-controlled dinner, such as Healthy Choice, if that works for you. Be sure that you get a chicken, turkey, or shrimp entrée with fewer than 300 total calories and less than 25 percent fat. I don't believe in getting the red meat choices, even in controlled-calorie frozen dinners, since you are trying to avoid red meat in your diet.

To achieve portion control in their own cooking, some of my patients save the divided dishes these dinners are packaged in. You can buy divided dishes in any kitchen supply store, and there are also disposable divided dishes. All of this can help you control portion size at dinner. You can be eating the right foods, but if you are eating extra large portions you will be working against yourself.

❏ *Use "friendly" take-out at home.* You've probably heard the old joke about the wife whose favorite recipe was reservations at a

Low-Fat Cooking for Different Foods

Learning how to cook the low-fat way is not difficult. You just need to know the best ways to prepare different ingredients.

Chicken Breasts

Buy precut, boneless chicken breast without skin, and try to find a supplier who uses no hormones or preservatives. Chicken breast is one of the most versatile protein items you can prepare. You can marinate it in a variety of sauces, including teriyaki marinade, Italian spices, Dijon mustard, and orange sauce. Serve with whole wheat pasta and tomato sauce, or with brown rice, whole wheat noodles, or potatoes. If you love to barbecue, chicken can be a great substitute for hamburger or steak. Just be careful of turkey burgers made with dark meat. They can derive up to 40 percent of their calories from fat, even though they are labeled 22 percent fat by weight.

If you want to have a barbecue regardless of the weather outside, and if you have a gas stove, you can buy a nonstick cooktop broiler. The fat from the chicken drops down into a stainless steel trough at the base. These devices usually cost about twenty dollars, and are easy to clean. Cook extra chicken breasts and refrigerate them for economical low-fat sandwiches the next day.

Shrimp

Shrimp can be broiled or barbecued on a skewer with red pepper, green pepper, and onion slices. You can grill shrimp with garlic or scallions, and put them over pasta or rice. You can also add shrimp to tomato sauce and garlic or mushrooms, and layer the sauce over pasta for a great gourmet meal. While shrimp is more expensive than other meats on a per-pound basis, you only need three to six small shrimp per person to meet the three- to six-ounce protein requirement at dinner.

Fish

Ahi tuna, swordfish, and halibut are great barbecued. You may need to get a special basket to keep the fish from falling apart over the barbecue. You can also broil fish indoors on an elevated grill to separate the fish from the fatty drippings. Add scallions, soy sauce, or teriyaki sauce for variety. If you are not a fish lover, flounder and sole are mild-flavored fish that can be marinated in any of the spices you would use for chicken. One of my favorite fish dishes is cioppino, or fisherman's stew. Simply put cut-up fish and tomato sauce with oregano, garlic, and other seasonings to taste in a big pot, and simmer. You can also add shrimp and scallops to make the cioppino restaurant style.

Vegetables

You get more nutrients if you don't boil nonstarchy vegetables in water. Steam vegetables such as broccoli, asparagus, or carrots in a double boiler or steamer. Or place a small amount of water in a microwave-safe dish, add the vegetables, and microwave for a few minutes. Don't add butter, cheese, fat, or oil. Instead, use rosemary, thyme, celery salt, dried onions, and dried garlic or garlic powder. Or squeeze half a fresh lemon over the cooked food. Try mixing different vegetables together for variety.

Potatoes are easy to bake in the microwave or oven. Add salsa, mustard, or plain nonfat yogurt as a sour cream substitute. Using beans and other legumes (peas, lentils, chickpeas, etc.) is a great way to add protein value to vegetarian dishes. Use equal amounts of legumes and either corn or rice to provide a balanced serving of protein. Approximately 1 cup of rice and 1 cup of beans is equivalent to a four-ounce serving of chicken in terms of protein. Be careful, though. When you add lots of beans to a meal, you also add significant calories.

Salads

Buy bagged greens that are already cut up. This eliminates the most labor-intensive part of making a salad. The dark green types, such as endive, chicory, and escarole, have more nutrients than watery iceberg lettuce. Some dark greens taste like licorice, while others have a slightly bitter taste. After the greens are in place, get a chopping board and go to town. Add green pepper, red pepper, mushrooms, carrots, alfalfa sprouts, and anything else you want—just don't add croutons or beans. (See page 68 for a list of good salad vegetables.) Use flavored vinegar instead of oil. You can buy rice vinegar in various flavors, red wine vinegars, or balsamic vinegar. If you are eating because of stress, having seconds on salad is a great idea.

Desserts

Cut-up melons, such as honeydew, cantaloupe, and watermelon, make a great summertime dessert. If available, add some grapes and chopped pineapple. In the winter, a nutless Waldorf salad, made with apples, pears, raisins, and cranberry juice, is terrific. The salad can also be cooked in the microwave and served warm.

Sorbets made from fruits such as strawberries or raspberries are easy summer treats. Just add some fruit and chopped ice to a blender. Blend until a slush forms, scoop the mixture into dishes, and place the dishes in the freezer. Serve with a sprig of mint.

local restaurant. Today it is possible to get lots of help and still look like a gourmet cook. There are take-out foods available from many restaurants. You can order the entrée, assuming it meets our Resolution Diet principles (see pages 120 to 125), and then add the vegetables and salad. When you serve at home, set up the dishes as if you were going out. You may want to buy new dishes for different seasons of the year to make it seem special when you are eating a meal at home. You will maintain control over your portion size and calories, and you will have the convenience of staying at home.

❑ *Leave the kitchen after dinner.* It's easy to snack if you are surrounded by food. So after dinner, leave the kitchen. If you are having another couple in for dinner, plan a special activity after the meal, such as walking in a mall or taking in a movie, so that you will not be tempted to snack all evening.

HOW TO EAT AT WORK

Throughout this country there are many families in which there are two wage earners. This means that more people than ever are eating at their workplaces, and often a healthy diet falls by the wayside.

Breakfast at Work

Breakfast at work is a high-risk situation because you're on the go and liable to grab an oily muffin or a buttered roll. Check out these strategies instead.

❑ *Make smart "eat-on-the-go" choices.* Do you leave home very early for a long commute to work? Do you get up just in time to catch the subway, train, or bus? If so, oftentimes you probably skip breakfast or just have a cup of coffee on the way out the door. If you don't have time for breakfast, take a ready-to-drink meal replacement, such as Ultra Slim-Fast, and a fruit with you. Once you get stuck in traffic or find your seat, you will have plenty of time to enjoy your breakfast while you listen to the radio or relax.

❏ *Take time to relax over breakfast at the workplace.* You can, of course, eat at your desk—just try not to dive right into work while doing so. The idea is to eat in a relaxed, unhurried manner. If your workplace has a microwave or a hot-water dispenser, you can even make oatmeal in the office. Just make a point of getting in a little early and taking some time for yourself before the day begins.

❏ *Beware of the coffee truck and the coffee house.* When you get to work, avoid the coffee truck. It is full of high-fat, high-calorie treats, such as doughnuts, coffee cakes, and rolls, along with the infamous cinnamon bun (which can have over 1,000 calories all by itself). If you don't have a coffeemaker in your office and can't convince your boss to spring for one, offer to share the costs of coffee supplies and a coffeemaker with some of your coworkers. You will all save money and avoid a high-risk situation by staying away from the coffee truck.

An upscale version of the coffee truck is the coffee house. (I still can't understand paying all that money for a caffe latte that costs pennies to make, but I guess you are paying for the atmosphere.) The coffee house, like its mobile cousin, has lots of tempting high-calorie treats. Coffees and iced drinks made with whipped cream and added sugar are now available as high-calorie coffee equivalents. Just have the plain coffee and pass on the other stuff.

❏ *Know what to eat at breakfast meetings.* If you are at a buffet breakfast, plan your eating. Have eggs poached or boiled with as little yellow as possible, or no yolk at all. Two to three eggs will provide you with adequate protein. Add some fruit and a piece of high-fiber wheat bread. A cup of coffee completes this breakfast. If you are still hungry, have a small bowl of high-fiber cereal with nonfat milk, but don't just keep eating. Declare an end to the meal and get rid of your silverware at some point.

Lunch at Work

Lunch offers a welcome respite from the daily routine, and is a time for relaxation with your coworkers. You just have to avoid the pitfalls that lunch brings.

❑ *Beware the business lunch.* If you have a business lunch scheduled, plan to have a meal replacement at your desk before lunch. You can order a large salad with a balsamic or wine vinegar dressing on the side, along with a glass of iced tea or a cup of coffee. That way, you won't be hungry, but you will have something to munch on while business is discussed. Watch out for bread or chips at the table; see page 119 for ways to avoid the bread basket. If you do order a more substantial meal, see pages 120 through 125 for advice on what to order in various types of restaurants, and remember to eat a lighter-than-usual dinner.

❑ *Pack a low-fat lunch.* You can, of course, bring in a bagged lunch; see page 111 for suggestions. If you want a warm lunch at work, you should make use of the office refrigerator and microwave. Bring in a frozen portion-controlled dinner and microwave your lunch. If you are working late, having an afternoon meal replacement on hand makes good sense to keep your energy levels high. Again, avoid buying food from coffee trucks or other food vendors who may come to the office.

❑ *Eat with people who eat sensibly, or eat alone.* Everyone wants to be sociable at the office, but that doesn't mean you should share the lunchroom with people who eat large amounts of food. The temptation will be too great. Find lunch companions who eat the way you do, or eat by yourself.

❑ *Use lunch hour for exercise, too.* My patients who have desk jobs often eat at their desks and then go out for a walk during the lunch hour. That's an excellent way to work exercise into your busy schedule.

Social Eating at Work

From time to time, people like to socialize at work. That's great, but there are situations you must plan for.

❏ *Become a birthday cake taster.* This is one of the key high-risk situations. For example, say someone is having a birthday. There's a big party. "Come on, have a piece of cake. Just this once." That's 500 calories of fat and sugar you don't need. Go to the party, but tell everyone that you are on a special program of tasting birthday cakes only. Then have one forkful, and that's it. You don't feel deprived and you don't insult anyone, but you don't accept your own 500-calorie serving on a plate. If you do, you know you will finish it. The same thing goes for birthday breakfasts, which often come complete with doughnuts, cookies, and other high-calorie foods. Have a corner of someone's special homemade brownie, but no more.

❏ *Plan for the holiday party season.* The run of December holiday parties is one long high-risk situation. Here you will usually find nuts, cheese, and wine, as well as cakes, to tempt you. I have developed a great strategy for this situation. First of all, get some sparkling water with a lime wedge in it. That will look like a drink. Find someone to talk to far away from the table of goodies. Circulate at this outside perimeter by either allowing one person to monopolize the conversation for the whole time or by working your way among the most talkative people you can find. In no time, the party will be over and you will have survived another high-risk situation.

❏ *Stay away from candy.* Two other hazards in the workplace are worth mentioning. One is the vending machine full of candy bars near the coffee machine. Standing and talking near vending machines can be dangerous if you indulge in a 400-calorie chocolate caramel nougat candy bar. Stay away from both the machine and the second hazard—the candy jar. In an effort to create a friendly environment, many workers put candy jars on their desks and fill them with sweets. Stay far away from these jars, since they can be land mines in your war against fat.

HOW TO EAT AWAY FROM HOME

Once you have removed all the high-risk foods from your pantry and mastered your eating at work, your greatest challenges will come outside of the home, whether it is eating at a restaurant, the homes of friends and relatives, or at night spots.

Overall Strategies for Eating at Restaurants

Eating out has become a form of entertainment for most of us. But there are ways to eat out and keep your resolution. Here are some general guidelines that can help you no matter where you choose to eat.

❏ *Don't leave the house hungry.* You should prepare for a meal out before you even leave home. Have some water and fiber or fruit, or at least some water by itself. Do not go out hungry—that will only lead you to make unwise choices.

❏ *Avoid the "freebees."* I did not list bread as a trigger food, but it, along with other premeal items as chips or cheese, can lead you to overeat while you are waiting for dinner to arrive. An alternative is to drink water while you are waiting, and ask the other members of your group if they don't mind not asking for bread or chips. If you ask, you may find that everyone is relieved to not have that bread basket at the table. If some people want bread, have the waiter bring out only one roll or slice for you, or simply put the basket near someone else. This is a tough high-risk situation, and you won't always succeed, but identify it every time and you will get better at controlling this source of extra calories.

❑ *Share, or shoot for leftovers.* Today's style in restaurants is to serve big portions on big plates—portion sizes in the United States are much larger than in most countries. If you are having dinner for two, think about sharing a higher-calorie entrée, and then having a large salad that you split. If you are eating alone, push aside the food you don't plan to eat and take it home in a doggy bag. Avoid ordering large or super-size portions just because they are more economical.

❑ *Ask the chef for help.* If you don't see any low-fat choices on the menu, ask. Ask for your vegetables steamed and your fish broiled. Also ask that your meal be made with as little oil or other cooking fat as possible. Have the kitchen hold the dressing, mayo, butter, cheese, and sour cream.

❑ *If the restaurant does not work with you, don't go back.* Always remember that you are the customer, so it's your wishes that count. If the restaurant makes it clear they don't like special orders, drop that establishment from your list.

Strategies for Different Types of Restaurants

You can get a low-fat dinner at almost any restaurant. The secret is knowing exactly which items to order, and which to avoid.

Fast Food

There are thousands of fast food restaurants in the United States. They are not ideal places to eat, but there will be times when fast food is the only choice available. If you have forgotten to carry a healthy snack, you will need the following survival skills.

❑ *Go for the low cal.* Your best choice is the broiled chicken breast sandwich. This type of sandwich is called a BK Broiler at Burger

King and a Broiled Chicken Sandwich at McDonald's. If you can get a garden salad with chicken breast, this is a good choice. Avoid eating too much salad dressing by dipping your fork in the dressing and then picking up your lettuce, rather than pouring the dressing on top of your salad. Finally, have a diet soda or iced tea to complete your meal. Never order a super-size anything.

❑ *Have it your way.* Have them hold the mayo, dressings, and cheese. They just add calories.

❑ *Remember that no fast food is good fast food.* My recommendation is that you avoid fast foods altogether. These places usually only carry low-fat (light) milk instead of fat-free milk. The deep-fried breaded chicken or fish are both loaded with oil. The fries sit under a heat lamp in all their greasy glory. And the burgers are a nutritional disaster. Fast food typifies what is wrong with American eating habits today. If you find yourself on the road and hungry, look for a cafeteria-style restaurant (see below) as a quick-meal alternative.

Cafeteria-Style Restaurants

If you are willing to pay just a bit more, you can get much better food than fast food from a new variety of prepared food restaurants that specialize in homecooked-style meals.

❑ *Know where to go, and what to order.* In terms of healthy and delicious food, one chain stands out above the rest. While not yet open in every part of the United States, Koo Koo Roo California Kitchens provides a flame-broiled chicken breast that has about 10 percent of its calories from fat. They have steamed vegetables and fresh salads. You will also find turkey breast that is only 5 percent fat.

❑ *Know what to avoid.* You still have to be careful in these some of these restaurants, though. Avoid ham and meatloaf, and higher-calorie side dishes, such as macaroni and cheese. That includes the Caesar salad, which is loaded with oil and cheese. Make sure you order white-meat chicken or turkey, and remove the skin.

❑ *Hold the high-fat extras.* Have them hold the mayo, butter, sour cream, dressings, and cheese. They just add calories.

Chinese Food

Chinese food in China is among the lowest-fat foods in the world. It is high in fiber and rich in soy protein. Unfortunately, restaurants serving Chinese food in the United States have succumbed to American temptation and now use fat in large amounts. As a result, Americanized Chinese food is among the highest-fat foods available.

❑ *Avoid fatty appetizers.* Pass up the high-fat egg rolls, spareribs, and fried wonton dishes as appetizers, and sip some green tea until the soup arrives.

❑ *Order the right soup.* Egg-drop soup is fairly low in fat. A bowl of hot-and-sour soup can be fairly low in fat, if it is thickened with rice or corn starch and has no added oil. If you're not sure, ask.

❑ *Choose your low-cal entrées.* Order steamed vegetables (broccoli, carrots, asparagus, etc.) and white rice (instead of fried rice). Then choose a dish made with Szechwan garlic sauce over white meat of chicken, shrimp, or scallops. Scallions add taste as well as healthy phytonutrients, substances believed to help prevent heart disease, cancer, and premature aging. Avoid dishes such as lemon chicken, Kung Pao chicken, crispy fish or chicken, egg foo young, orange duck or beef, and Hunan shredded pork.

❑ *Ask the waiter for help.* Many times Chinese sauces or syrups contain tons of calories. Have them hold the sauce or serve it on the side. Substitute steamed vegetables for the oil-cooked version in your order. Ask if they can use dried chili peppers instead of hot oil to provide that fiery spark, or ask for hot mustard sauce. Have them hold the nuts and sweetened fruits.

Italian and Greek Food

The traditional Mediterranean diets of Italy and Greece have a great reputation, since Italy and Greece had among the lowest rates of cancer and heart disease in the 1960s. This is where olive oil got its great reputation as the healthiest salad and cooking oil. Today, there are pizzas in which cheese is stuffed into the crust. In many Italian and Greek restaurants, oil is added to many traditional dishes.

❑ *Learn to eat light Italian style.* To eat light at an Italian restaurant, order the traditional Italian family salad (not the antipasto) with balsamic vinegar (no oil). Have no more than one slice of Italian bread (not cheesy garlic bread). Stay away, obviously, from the fried calamari and fried mozzarella cheese, and the creamy or cheesy entrées. Order pasta with marinara sauce or a pasta primavera to which steamed vegetables have been added.

❑ *Go Greek the low-cal way.* Greek salad is very similar to Italian salad, except it is usually made with feta cheese. Ask the waiter to leave out the cheese. Beyond the salad, you have a problem. The lamb used for gyros is high in fat, so you may want to look for a white-meat chicken dish or a fish dish, preferably baked. If there is a vegetarian dish without cheese, that could be a good choice. You can look for dishes made with orzo, a ricelike pasta, that have no meat or cheese. Obviously, this isn't easy. If it's a special occasion, cut down on the high-fat main dish and have double helpings of salad and vegetables.

❑ *Split your meal and cut the calories in half.* Split the pasta or orzo, meat, and salad with a companion—usually the portions are large enough for two. This sharing policy not only cuts down on the size of the bill, but will cut the number of calories you consume. Pasta can make you overfat if you eat enough of it, especially since most pasta in restaurants is made from refined flour with most of its fiber removed.

❏ *Ask the waiter for help.* Request that your food be prepared with as little oil as possible. Ask for the dressing on the side. Have them hold the butter, the oil, and in Greek restaurants, the pita with yogurt dipping sauce. Also, in Italian restaurants, go easy on the Parmesan cheese—it's very flavorful in small amounts. If the cheese shaker is a temptation, have the waiter take it away after you're finished with it.

Japanese Food

There are some great choices available in Japanese restaurants, which generally carry a lot of low-fat items on their menus.

❏ *Go easy on the sushi.* When you are eating sushi, have the equivalent of 3 to 6 ounces of raw fish and 1 cup of rice. Then you can have some vegetables and salad or a cup of miso soup to round out your meal. Some people overeat sushi. Even though sushi is low in fat, if you eat these delicious finger foods until you are full, you will get way too many calories.

❏ *Choose low-fat entrées.* Teriyaki made with white-meat chicken or shrimp is fine. So is the yakatori, or broiled chicken kabobs. Have the udon (wheat) or soba (buckwheat) noodles—they are among the few whole-grain noodles you will find as standard fare in restaurants. Be sure to avoid all tempura dishes, since they are deep-fried.

❏ *Ask the waiter for help.* Ask for wasabe mustard (careful, it's really hot) or for the pickled ginger that generally comes with sushi. Have them serve other sauces on the side. Substitute steamed vegetables for the oil-cooked version in your order.

Mexican Food

Like Chinese food, Mexican food became a high-fat cuisine when it came to the United States. There is fat everywhere on the plate, especially since shredded cheddar cheese and sour cream are used as garnishes.

❑ *Be careful at the bar*. Margaritas are among the highest-calorie drinks, delivering up to 350 calories per drink. If you want a drink, a light beer with a slice of lemon is a good choice, and sparkling water with lime is even better.

❑ *Stick with light starters*. Ceviche is an interesting alternative to nachos. This is an appetizer made with seafood marinated in vinegar. Gazpacho, a chilled soup made with tomatoes and cucumbers, is another good opener.

❑ *Order a low-fat entrée*. I usually order a chicken, fish, or shrimp tostada. I eat the meat and the lettuce. I will have some of the beans and pass on the cheese and the high-fat taco shell. Try the grilled chicken and fish items. Chicken, shrimp, or vegetable fajitas are OK, as long as you have the corn tortillas instead of the flour, and if you split the dish with someone. Avoid the fried items, and also avoid the Mexican rice, which is often cooked with lard.

❑ *Ask the waiter for help*. Ask whether or not the beans are fried in lard, and whether or not you can get whole black beans instead of refried beans. Have them hold the sour cream, guacamole, and cheese, and ask for extra salsa, verde sauce, or tomatillo sauce.

Eating at the Homes of Friends and Relatives

It's always good to spend time with family and friends. But such get-togethers can present high-risk situations.

❑ *Flatter the family baker—without giving in to temptation.* Major family holidays—Thanksgiving, Christmas or Hanukkah, birthdays, anniversaries—can present high-risk situations, especially when you are asked to eat the host's favorite dish. For example, you are at Aunt Bertha's house, and she brings out her famous cheesecake. This is the one that made her the most famous baker in town. It is only about 700 calories per slice, and here comes Aunt Bertha with a big piece just for you. Your best choice is to tell her you will just have a taste to confirm how great it is for everyone within earshot to hear, and then to take just a forkful. Don't put the whole piece of cake on your plate, just the taste. If you really want to be polite, just take an extremely thin sliver-slice. If you are not that close to Aunt Bertha, then simply tell her you remember how great her cheesecake was but you just can't afford to eat that way any more. If she insists, tell her your doctor instructed you to stay away from cheesecake.

❑ *Remember portion control.* When food is getting passed around the table at big family dinners, think about what you are taking as your portion. This is one time you get to practice portion control. At Thanksgiving, I have 3 to 6 ounces of turkey (pieces one to two times the size of the palm of my hand), 1 cup of steamed carrots, and half of a small baked potato. I have salad with balsamic vinegar or wine vinegar on the side. I have coffee but no pumpkin pie for dessert. If there is cut-up fruit, I will have that.

❑ *Get away from the dinner table.* As soon as possible after Thanksgiving meal, I leave the table and either head out to the backyard or to the local TV set tuned to some regional football rivalry. I have sparkling water with lime as I talk to relatives and friends, and stay away from any high-calorie goodies that may be available. (I'll maybe take a pretzel or two.) I always slightly pat myself on the back for having survived another high-risk holiday situation.

❑ *Offer to bring a low-fat dish.* One way to avoid temptation when eating at someone else's house is to call before you go and ask if you can bring anything with you. Then offer to prepare a low-calorie dish for the communal table, and eat most of your meal out of that.

Eating at Weddings, Reunions, Nightspots, and Dance Clubs

It's the big night, and you're all dressed up and ready to go. But don't forget your resolution.

❑ *Eat before you go, and watch what you eat when you get there.* Weddings, reunions, and other celebrations, including New Year's Eve, are gala events where everyone is dressed to the hilt and where rich dishes such as salmon, steak, chicken stuffed with cheese, and rich desserts are served. My approach is to eat a protein entrée or a meal replacement, such as Ultra Slim-Fast, before I go to the event. Then when I am there, I will have the salad, the vegetables, a little rice, and lots of water. I stay away from desserts altogether. I have decaffeinated coffee as the evening draws to a close, and what's more, I do not feel deprived. Rather I feel that I have overcome another high-risk situation.

❑ *Know what to order from the bar.* At nightspots and dance clubs, you can drink sparkling water with a lime wedge for appearance's sake. If you are going to have some alcohol, the lowest-calorie choices are wine or beer. Stay away from margaritas or sweetened cocktails. Also avoid chips, crackers, cheese, nuts, and other treats left around the bar.

❑ *Remember that dancing is exercise, too.* Get into fast dancing. The more you dance, the more fat you burn. It is a great activity for maintaining your fitness and burning off fat.

Practical strategies only work if you practice them every day. What are your most common problems? We live in what I believe is a toxic nutritional environment—a sea of fat and sugar. You can take control of your environment and succeed, without feeling deprived. You won't need to be perfect, and you should not expect to be perfect. Just put as many of these strategies as you can into practice, and you will be able to master the trigger situation strategy as well as the trigger food strategy as part of the Resolution Diet. In the next chapter, I will show you how exercise makes it easier to keep your resolution.

Your Personal Everyday-Eating
PROFILE

Answer the following eleven questions to determine how you can avoid high-calorie situations every day.

IDENTIFYING HIGH-RISK SITUATIONS

1. What are your high-risk situations in the kitchen?

2. What are your high-risk situations at work?

3. What are your high-risk situations in restaurants?

4. What are your high-risk situations at special occasions?

5. What are your high-risk situations at nightspots or
dance clubs?

6. What are your favorite restaurants?
☐ Fast food   ☐ American   ☐ Chinese
☐ Italian   ☐ Greek   ☐ Mexican
☐ Other:_____

REDUCING YOUR RISK

7. What are the most important things you could do to reduce
your fat and sweet intake at your favorite restaurant?

8. What are two recipes you would like to make at home?

9. How could you modify these recipes to reduce fat and sugar?

10. How could you control the portion sizes of foods at dinner?

11. Are there after-dinner eating habits you could control?

Chapter 7

Get the Exercise and Stress-Reduction Habits

E ating properly is a good habit. But it won't do you any good if you don't develop the other key habit: exercise. Keeping weight off over the long term requires regular exercise, along with just generally getting off the couch and becoming more active whenever you can in your daily life. As with our eating habits, our lifestyles have become so sedentary that they represent a threat to our health. Not only is exercise a great way to burn fat and adjust your metabolism, but it is also a great stress reducer and a natural antidepressant.

The ability of exercise to combat stress is important, because every day I talk to patients who overeat out of stress. We all have stress in our lives from all sorts of sources. That makes learning to deal with stress another important habit. While exercise is the most potent antidote I know to our stressful lifestyles, it works hand in hand with other methods of reducing stress.

In this chapter, I am going to help you to achieve your exercise and stress-relief potential. First, I'll explain why exercise is so important and how your muscles work. Then I will discuss the importance of stretching to maintain flexibility and posture. I will show you how to burn fat, and how to tone your heart and circulation, through aerobic exercise. I will teach you the principles of muscle building, and how this can increase your metabolism so that you burn even more fat. I will also give you ways to fit exercise into your everyday activities. Finally, I will pay a closer look at the issue of stress. You will plan your personal exercise and stress-reduction program using the profile at the end of the chapter.

WHY EXERCISE?

Surfing the Internet is *not* a sport. Your body is designed for a high level of physical activity. Exercise, like a desire for sweet, fatty foods, was programmed into our ancestors, whose lives were full of hard physical labor. And just as the modern diet has swamped the body's appetite center, so too has forced inactivity overwhelmed the body's built-in desire for movement. Many of us spend our days in front of the computer and our evenings in front of the TV. Neither activity burns many calories. The idea is to match your physical activity genes (yes, you do have some!) to leisure-time physical activities and some formal customized exercises so that you can reach your full potential for a healthy weight and a vigorous metabolism. In addition, exercise helps build healthy bones. This helps prevent osteoporosis in later life, a condition in which the bones become porous and brittle.

The other main reason to exercise is because it helps keep stress at bay—it really does lift your spirits. I have sometimes been so tired that I just couldn't face going to the gym for a workout. But once I was there working out on an exercise cycle, my mood built and I would have one of my best workouts ever. This was not just my imagination. Exercise releases chemicals called endorphins, which influence the pleasure center in your brain. You literally become addicted to the feeling of a good workout. Exercise can be an important tool in combating so-called burn-out depression, which is the most common form of depression. When you exercise, especially outdoors, your brain's own chemicals help fight the blue feelings. (I have had friends who have taken up jogging after painful divorces, and claim to this day that the habit saved them.) And as we've seen in previous chapters, stress is a common reason for overeating.

You often hear people complain that they are exercising, but not losing weight. ("Why should I bother exercising?") It is important to realize that burning fat through exercise involves both a short-term and a longer-term strategy. In the short term, aerobic exercise is the key. Walking at a slow, comfortable pace is, surprisingly, the best and most efficient way to burn fat. When walking at a slow rate, 60 percent of the total energy being burned is from your body's fat stores. Since you can walk for a longer period at a slow rate, you can burn a lot more fat than if you become quickly exhausted at a full run or rapid walk. The longer-term strategy for burning fat is to perform activities that build muscle, called anaerobic exercise. This will require six months to a year of work, and will need to be done independently of your aerobic exercise.

The best single answer to the question, "Why exercise?" is this: the one behavior that correlates best with maintaining weight loss is burning more than 2,000 calories per week. That's about 300 calories a day. Making exercise a regular habit pays off.

HOW MUSCLES WORK

Knowing something about how your muscles work will help you in your workouts. Your muscles are connected intimately to your brain by millions of nerves. When the nerve sends an electrical signal to the muscle, that signal releases a trigger mechanism, which keeps the muscle's fibers apart. They spring together so that they overlap, and when this process is duplicated simultaneously by thousands of muscle fibers, you get a muscle contraction. After the contraction is over, your muscle cell must take up energy to reset the trigger mechanism. So the actual contraction doesn't require energy, but resetting the muscle does.

It is important to realize this because after heavy exercise, you must nourish your muscles. Eating some carbohydrate and protein after exercise gives your muscles the energy they need to prepare for the next round of exercise. Athletes who are kept from eating in exercise experiments can only perform at a fraction of their usual ability after just a few hours of starvation. Today, many athletes take nutrition and fluids while they are exercising to maintain their endurance. The muscles are designed to burn fat when they exercise.

The muscles also take up a lot of carbohydrate as sugar from the bloodstream. If you are usually inactive, your muscles are smaller and less able to burn sugar or fat for energy, so you become an efficient fat storage machine. So muscles have two functions. First, they have a contracting function, which allows us to move and be active. Second, they have a calorie-burning function, which burns any extra food we eat during and after exercise.

We have two kinds of muscles. The smooth muscles in the heart and intestines contract without our knowing it. We can exercise them by eating more fiber or doing aerobic training. Conscious muscle training involves the skeletal muscles, which move when you want them to. If you decide to move your finger across this page, you don't need to think about each movement. Your finger, hand, and arm are perfectly coordinated. This level of coordination, though, pales by comparison to the hand-eye coordination of a baseball pitcher throwing a fastball at 100 miles per hour. The muscles in our bodies are able to evolve and shape their functions to the activities we participate in. So a golfer, a long-distance runner, a sprinter, a sculptor, and a concert pianist each have differently developed muscles that are highly specialized to the tasks they have been repeating for years and years.

Within each muscle bundle there are fibers specialized for either strength or endurance. These are generally called white and red muscle. A chicken breast is white muscle adapted to contracting rapidly and repeatedly to beat the chicken's wings. The dark meat of the legs is red muscle able to support the weight of the chicken's body over long periods of time. This muscle is adapted to endurance rather than speed and strength.

In fact, all skeletal muscles have a mixture of these different types of fibers. Which type develops depends on the functions you want your muscles to perform. For example, the muscles in the lower back must retain contractions for long periods to retain posture, while your finger muscles move quickly in typing or other fine motor tasks.

How do muscles shape and rebuild themselves for these different tasks? This process occurs through injury of the muscle when it is overstressed. When the muscle is extended and before it contracts, you can injure the muscle cells by stretching them. When this happens, signals are sent to other muscle cells that grow and fuse with the damaged cells, enlarging and strengthening them with more fibers. This process is similar to what happens in a long bone after a fracture, in which a section of thicker, stronger bone grows over the fracture site. Similarly, in muscle the injury leaves the muscle stronger and bigger.

STRETCHING TO GET READY FOR EXERCISE

You should always stretch before beginning any type of exercise. You need to stretch so that the weaker muscles can get out of the cramped positions they assumed during periods of inactivity. Stretching will also increase blood flow to the muscles and will increase the temperature of the tendons the muscles are attached to, making it less likely the muscles will be pulled to the point of injury during exercise. Stretching is also a great stress reducer. Much of the nervous tension of the day can be stored in the muscles of the neck and shoulders.

Stretching is only useful if it is done properly. Make sure you stretch all the major muscle groups in your legs, arms, chest, and back. Be sure to hold each stretch for about ten seconds before moving onto the next muscle group. Do not move sharply and quickly; slow, gentle movements are best. Breathe naturally and easily during stretching—don't hold your breath. If you are exercising outside in cold weather, make sure you stretch for a longer period of time than you do in warmer weather. It's also a good idea in cold weather to warm up a little before stretching. Running in place or doing some jumping jacks will help you avoid injury.

BURNING CALORIES THROUGH AEROBIC EXERCISE

During aerobic exercise, your muscles will become more attuned to burning fat, and they will increase their fat-burning activity even at rest. In addition to burning fat, regular exercise will help keep your cardiovascular system in peak operating condition. It's also a good idea to do some aerobic exercise before lifting weights. By exercising your muscles, you will be increasing the blood flow to muscles, tendons, and joints. This reduces the chance of injury during weightlifting.

You should run, walk, cycle, or swim at a rate at which you can comfortably carry on a conversation. The heart rate that allows you to do this is called the target heart rate; see "Calculating Your Target Heart Rate" on the next page.

Your workouts can be done up to seven days per week, and should take from thirty to forty minutes a session. Simply work up to your target rate during a ten-minute warmup, maintain your target rate for twenty minutes, and cool down for another ten minutes. You can do this on a treadmill or cycle while watching television. Try to do this every day if you can, but if you can only manage five out of seven days, that's fine.

Remember, exercise needs to be enjoyable. That way, you will always look forward to it, and it will remain an exciting and stimulating part of your daily activities. Another way to increase your aerobic fitness is to take a full day out for cycling or hiking on a weekend. You will feel the positive, relaxing effects of this exercise for a full day after your high-activity outing.

BUILDING MUSCLES THROUGH HEAVY RESISTANCE EXERCISE

Building muscle is important for two reasons. First, each pound

Calculating Your Target Heart Rate

The target heart rate is the rate at which your heart is beating fast enough to become stronger by creating positive changes in the heart muscle. You can easily check your own heart rate by placing a finger on the carotid artery in your neck. That's the one you can feel beating near your windpipe. Just count the number of beats for fifteen seconds and multiply by four.

Before calculating your target rate, you should check your resting heart rate. Check your resting rate after a full night's sleep, before you get out of bed. The faster the rate, the harder your heart has to work even before you start doing anything. Over time, your resting rate will drop as you become more physically fit.

You can calculate your target rate as follows:

1. Start by subtracting your age from the number 220. This is called your maximum heart rate (MHR):

$$220 - age = MHR$$

2. You now want to determine your initial target heart rate (ITHR). This is the heart rate you want to aim for during the first six weeks of your exercise program:

$$MHR \times .5 \text{ to } .6 = ITHR$$

3. After six weeks, your heart will be in better condition. You can then set your conditioned target heart rate (CTHR):

$$MHR \times .7 \text{ to } .8 = CTHR$$

For example, if you are fifty, your MHR is 170 and your ITHR would be 85 to 102 beats per minute. After you are accustomed to exercise, you can raise your exercise intensity to the CTHR, which would be 119 to 136 beats per minute. Always stay within these ranges, except when you are warming up and cooling down from exercise. If you drop below 50 percent of your maximum heart rate, you will be spending more time exercising than you need to while giving your heart less of a workout than it would like. Anything over 80 percent of the maximum rate is too intense. So stay within the appropriate range.

of muscle burns 14 calories per day. That doesn't sound like much, but adding 20 pounds of muscle can add almost 300 calories to the number of calories you burn every day. This will allow you to eat more while maintaining your current body weight or, if you prefer, you can lose body fat more quickly. Second, muscle has an enzyme, called lipoprotein lipase, that burns fat. At a low level of exercise (50 to 70 percent of your maximum heart rate), 60 percent of the calories you burn are from fat. Low-level exercise burns the most fat, while at higher levels of exercise you burn relatively more carbohydrates. Also, the more muscle you have and the better conditioned that muscle is, the more fat you burn.

In order to build muscle, you must carefully stress the muscle. This will cause microscopic damage to the muscle fiber, but as we've seen, the muscle will super-compensate and become stronger as a result. The key to building muscle is to exercise enough to create this damage, and then to rest long enough to allow the muscle to rebuild and grow. This recovery period is when the muscle is built, and most weight-training coaches stress the importance of maximizing the recovery period. Typically, the same muscle groups are not exercised over and over again every day to exhaustion. That leads to breakdown of muscle fibers from overtraining.

It is important to select exercises that work both the agonistic and antagonistic muscles at each joint. These are muscles that work in opposition to each other, such as the biceps and triceps. (When the biceps are contracted, the triceps are stretched, and vice versa.) Every muscle builder wants a strong biceps. This is the large muscle you point to when you flex your arm. On the underside of your arm, though, you have the much-less-heralded triceps muscle. The triceps balances the work of the biceps, and is primarily responsible for movements such as pushing a weight up and away from your body. You cannot build strength effectively without building both the triceps and the biceps. This is a general principle of muscle building. Building both muscles in a pair balances the associated joint and prevents injury.

It is also important to balance the time devoted to building strength and endurance in each muscle group. The damage occurs when the muscle is stretched, so it is important to do your exercises carefully and spend adequate time in the stretching as well as contracting parts of each exercise. This can be accomplished by varying the number of sets of each exercise from three to seven, and varying the repetitions (reps) from eight to fifteen. (A repetition is one complete movement, from start to finish, and a set is a group of repetitions.) You should also vary the pace of the exercise, starting out at four to six seconds per repetition, and speeding it up to two to three seconds per repetition while using higher weights and fewer repetitions. It is best to get some instruction from a knowledgeable trainer. If you have any physical problems, see your doctor before you start training.

Be sure to make a written plan for the exercises you plan to pursue. You can take the profile at the back of this chapter to a trainer or physical therapist to get a set of written exercises. Weight training with dumbbells requires some instruction or experience. If you want to take the responsibility or cannot afford instruction, you can get a number of books and magazines with information on how to exercise. If you develop your own workout from magazines, be sure to do the movements correctly. Also pay attention to balancing your workout so that it includes the arms, chest, back, abdomen, and legs.

The most important thing when building muscle is to not get discouraged. This is a gradual process that takes many months. Follow the sample schedule I have developed to gradually work your way into muscle building.

Your First Visit

Get used to going to the gym. Play around with the equipment you plan to use. Don't worry about making progress. Always ask a knowledgeable trainer how to use the various machines and exercise equipment at your gym. On your own, you might injure yourself or get discouraged.

Week 1

Three sets of fifteen reps per exercise. If you cannot do this number of reps, then reduce the weight until you can. You should rest thirty seconds between exercises. Also, don't jerk the weights rapidly. Instead, spend four to six seconds per rep. Mentally concentrate on the muscles you are using to get the maximum benefit.

Week 2

Increase to five sets of fifteen reps per exercise. The last four reps of each set should cause some burning in the muscle groups.

Week 3

Increase to seven sets of fifteen reps per exercise.

Week 4

Decrease to three sets of twelve reps per exercise, but increase the weight. This way, you give the maximum stimulus to your muscles.

Week 5

Do five sets of twelve reps per exercise at the higher weight.

Week 6

Do seven sets of twelve reps per exercise at the higher weight.

Week 7

Do three sets of eight reps per exercise, but increase the weight again to get the maximum benefit. Do each rep for two to three seconds, and rest forty-five seconds between exercises.

Week 8

Do five sets of eight reps per exercise at the new weight.

Week 9

Do seven sets of eight reps per exercise at the new weight.

FITTING IN FITNESS FOR THE HARD-CORE COUCH POTATO

All right. I know you think exercise is actually a four-letter word. Your memories of running laps and doing jumping jacks in the cold air in high school won't go away. The sedentary society in which we live doesn't help. We literally drive to the elevator in this country, and park as close to the mall as we can. In short, as a society we have failed to organize our physical environment to encourage normal physical activity, much less regular exercise.

You may be able to find lots of ways to fit aerobic exercise into your daily schedule with some of the activities listed below, from least intense at the top to the most intense at the bottom:

- Gardening for thirty to forty-five minutes
- Washing windows or mopping floors for forty-five minutes
- Walking two miles in forty minutes
- Shooting baskets for thirty minutes
- Bicycling five miles in thirty minutes
- Dancing quickly (social dancing) for thirty minutes
- Pushing a baby in a stroller one and a half miles in thirty minutes
- Raking leaves for thirty minutes
- Walking two miles in thirty minutes

- Swimming laps for twenty minutes
- Playing basketball for fifteen to twenty minutes
- Bicycling four miles in fifteen minutes
- Jumping rope for fifteen minutes

What counts for cardiovascular conditioning is the total amount of activity. So you can choose to do something less intense for a longer period, or something more intense for a shorter period. In terms of burning fat, there is an advantage to doing the less intense activities for a longer period of time.

You've seen the ads for treadmills and weights and exercise machines of every description. They don't benefit you by simply collecting dust. You have to use them and any other method you can think of to get adequate exercise.

YOUR PERSONAL EXERCISE RESOLUTION

Exercise goals are as personalized as eating habits, and just as important. They must be tailored to your desires, abilities, and overall health and fitness needs. It is a mistake to copy your best friend's routine unless it happens to fit you perfectly. Also, the mental side of exercise is every bit as important as the physical side. You will need to draw on the same skills you are using to change your eating habits. Make a plan, and carry it out.

To accomplish your weight-loss goal, you need to create your own exercise target, just as you set a target weight in Chapter 2. The first step is to write down your top three fitness goals on the profile that follows. Ask yourself whether your most important objective is feeling healthy, losing weight, or developing your appearance. Visualizing your goals will help you allocate the time during each workout to stretching, aerobic, and weightlifting activities. It will take time to get used to this routine, but eventually you will feel great.

Don't forget to reward yourself as you go along. Get yourself a jogging outfit or some other gym equipment (perhaps a fancy water bottle or Walkman radio?) as you reach each new target, such as getting to the gym regularly, accomplishing your aerobic goals every time, starting your weight program, reaching some fitness goals, and so forth.

CONTROL STRESS: IT'S NOT WHAT YOU'RE EATING, BUT WHAT'S EATING YOU

Some stress is good. Stress provides us with the ability to be alert to danger and to flee when necessary. It stimulates us and gives us something to look forward to each day. Great actors and actresses will tell you that when they are nervous they give their best performances. No stress can actually be stressful. Yet while a certain level of stress is good, most of us have excessive levels of stress. Ultimately, this continuing stress can lead to the most common form of depression, called burn-out depression.

Face it! We live in a high-stress society. If we are to survive our modern-day saber-toothed tigers, we need to adapt. For years, I have been telling my patients about *The Seven Habits of Highly Effective People* by Steven Covey, and his more recent work, *First Things First*. These books contain principles that can help you define what your goals are, and how you want to achieve these goals. Often, stress is the result of not prioritizing the tasks in your daily life. Once you know your mission in life, you can prioritize those things that are most important and most urgent. Then you will learn to be in control of your own life, instead of giving that control to others. A complete discussion of Covey's aforementioned books is beyond the scope of this chapter, but I recommend that you read them and use them daily to order your life.

When you are in control, the stress you feel will not take its terrible toll. There is a famous experiment I first heard about in my college psychology class. There were two monkeys. One was given food every time he pressed a lever after a green light went off. He got an electrical shock every time he pressed the lever after a red light flashed. The green and red lights went off in a predictable way, and the monkey soon learned which lever to push. The other monkey was given a random sequence of green and red lights when each of the two levers was pushed. It was impossible to learn, and the poor monkey ultimately got a stress ulcer trying to figure it out.

So we know that stress is harmful, and that it can lead to overeating. How do you counteract stress? Well, exercise, as we've seen, is an important part of the solution. But there are other methods that will help you fight the stress that can lead you to eat.

DEVELOP STRATEGIES FOR REDUCING STRESS

There is no question that our society is more stressful today than ever. Uncontrollable stresses that affect important areas of life, such as a layoff threat or an ill parent, are particularly upsetting.

In some cases, you can try to look at the source of your stress in a different light. It has been said that life is a series of golden opportunities cleverly disguised as insurmountable problems. Anything facing you can be a great opportunity rather than a stressor. I recently met an engineer who was laid off during the defense cutbacks. He started his own business rather than looking for a job in engineering. After several tries, he founded an import-export business that has been very successful. He could have despaired, but instead he took stock of what he could do, and tried his best. Things don't always go well in life, but planning to succeed and working hard is a great stress reducer. In fact, Albert Einstein went so far as to say that hard work was a cure for worry-driven stress.

What if you are a hard worker who is overstressed? The first step to reducing stress is to realize that it is your reaction to stressful situations that is the problem. Let's say you are stuck in a traffic jam. You can lurch forward and slam the brakes every couple of minutes, or you can resign yourself to the fact that you are going to be stuck and put some quiet music on the radio instead of the news and traffic report updates (unless you need them). I often see patients who have serious disabilities to which they adjust and others who are stressed out by minor problems. Stress only has the power over you that you give it.

The next step in taking control over stress is to give yourself one day a week off to relax. It's an old idea called the Sabbath day, and it works. Remember when all the stores were closed on Sunday, and you rested at home instead of running off to the mall? Life was slower then. Fill your time instead with pleasure reading, listening to your favorite music, or just napping and relaxing. Tell yourself that you actually are doing important work—the work of refreshing yourself for the following week's tasks.

If, between work and other commitments, you can't take a whole day off, start with just an afternoon. Does this sound similar to our strategies for targeting certain foods to avoid? You're right! The principle is the same. You can be addicted to stress just as much as to high-fat foods. After all, there is status associated with being busy. So why not accept doing 80 to 90 percent of your tasks, as you do with your diet? You may find that the stress dissipates if you focus on the top 80 or 90 percent of your priorities and drop the bottom 10 to 20 percent.

If you take time off but are still troubled by stress, there are a number of stress-reduction techniques you can use, from deep breathing to biofeedback and mediation. Stress-reduction courses may be offered at your local high school or college in the evenings, or at other community centers such as the Y or the library. Finally, you should be aware that your problem with stress may be a sign of an underlying psychological problem, such as depression. If you think you have a problem, talk to your doctor.

Get Your Zzz's

Many people in our society are in an almost constant state of sleep deprivation. That's not good, because sleep provides stress reduction, especially when you get the deep sleep that is signaled by rapid eye movements (REM) under your eyelids. This happens about 2 A.M. for most people. If you have had a good night's sleep, you awaken refreshed. If you haven't, you are tired the whole day. This makes you irritable and fatigued, setting up a high-risk situation for binge eating in an attempt to feel better.

For some people, getting to sleep itself requires stress reduction, and some people love to have milk and cookies at night. Some of my patients can't get to sleep without this high-calorie aid. In most cases, they are settling their stress, which they feel in their stomachs. Instead of starting to relax in the fifteen minutes or even hour before bed, you should consider making your whole night more relaxing. A warm shower can relax tightened muscles, as can a session of stretching. Some quiet music and good conversation with friends is a great way to unwind. If catching up on your work at night is essential, stop at a fixed time each night. Make sure you have at least a couple of hours to relax.

You should be aware that there are some physical conditions, such as a breathing disorder called sleep apnea, that can make it difficult to get a good night's rest. Talk to your doctor if you have ongoing sleep problems.

Planning for High-Stress Situations

There are a lot of different ways people deal with stress, and eating is one of them. Sometimes the problem is behavioral, as in binge eating. Binge eating is an uncontrolled behavior that is rewarding while it is going on at some conscious or unconscious level, but often results in overwhelming guilt after the fact. How does this happen? You know that the binge eating behavior is something you want to avoid. It is an example of a chain of behaviors that ultimately can lead to uncontrollable eating.

The way to prevent this behavior is to break the chain of behaviors. For example, you might notice that a particular stressful situation leads to overeating. By planning for the situation carefully, you can break the chain. You may initially notice an environment that could lead to binge eating. This is the point at which you practice self-talk ("I am not going to eat that high-fat dessert they are bringing to the table"), or remove yourself from the high-risk environment (stand further away from the dessert table at a party). You then practice stimulus control by substituting something for the less healthy alternative ("Thanks, but I will just have coffee instead"). Finally, you should allow yourself to feel morally superior for having avoided your impulse to binge eat. That's right, mentally pat yourself on the back. The trick is to look like you are depriving yourself while not feeling deprived. When you can practice this entire chain of behaviors, it replaces the behaviors that lead to uncontrolled binge eating.

Now that you have reduced your binge-eating risk by dealing with your everyday stress, become conscious of stress-eating triggers and nip them in the bud. Every time you binge eat, write down the stress factor that set you off. Then you can plan to avoid these stressors whenever possible.

Make up your mind that you are going to go and exercise. Start slowly, but begin your exercise program soon. Realize that muscle building is a long-term goal, but aerobic exercise will get you burning calories right away. It will also condition your heart. Make a plan and get the advice you need, and you can build muscle at any age. The same thing goes for stress relief. Don't keep putting it off. Remember, the more stress you're under, the more likely you are to seek out trigger foods for comfort. In the next chapter, I will give you advice on how to stay focused on your resolutions.

Your Exercise and Stress-Reduction
PROFILE

Answer the following fifteen questions to determine how you can achieve your exercise and stress-reduction goals. Then follow the instructions on the separate sheet at the end.

SETTING YOUR EXERCISE GOALS

1. How would you describe your current level of physical activity?

   ☐ very active   ☐ moderately active   ☐ not very active
   ☐ completely sedentary (desk job with no physical activity)

2. Do you participate regularly in a sport or other physical activity now? What is it?

3. What are your top three exercise goals? (Examples: firm and shape; reduce weight; bodybuilding; strengthening; rehabilitation; general health)

   _____

   _____

   _____

GETTING MEDICAL CLEARANCE

4. Do you have any medical or physical condition which restricts your ability to exercise (knee pain, back pain, etc.)?

5. Have you seen your doctor for clearance before you start exercising?

CHOOSING THE BEST TIME TO EXERCISE

6. What time of the day is most convenient for you to exercise?

☐ AM   ☐ PM

7. What time interval can you commit to? (Plan to lift weights at least three days a week, but to walk thirty minutes every day.)

☐ 6–8 AM   ☐ 8–10 AM   ☐ 10AM–12PM   ☐ 12–2 PM
☐ 2–4 PM   ☐ 4–6 PM   ☐ 6–8 PM   ☐ 8–10 PM
☐ Other:_____

8. What are your three best days and times for exercise, including an alternate for each?

First Choice Days and Times   **Back-up Times/Days**

_____   _____

_____   _____

_____   _____

SELECTING THE BEST WAYS TO EXERCISE

9. What are your favorite forms of exercise?

10. What are your favorite leisuretime activities?

FINDING WAYS OF REDUCING STRESS

11. Name the three biggest sources of stress in your life.

_____

_____

_____

12. Reread question 7. What is the best day and time for you to take time for yourself?

13. Do you get enough sleep?

☐ Yes   ☐ No

14. If the answer is no, why don't you get enough sleep?

15. What are three other stress-reduction methods you can try? (Examples: meditation; biofeedback; tai chi; breathing exercises)

Exercise Record

Copy this on a separate sheet, and make multiple copies. Take a sheet with you to the gym, and fill out a new sheet every time you set new goals for yourself.

STRETCHING

1. How long do you plan to stretch each muscle group?

   Legs　　　　_____

   Arms　　　　_____

   Back　　　　_____

   Abdomen　　_____

   Chest　　　　_____

AEROBIC EXERCISE

2. My Target Heart Rate for thirty minutes is:_____

3. Record how you achieved this goal.

	Minutes	Heart Rate Achieved
Treadmill:	_____	_____
Walking:	_____	_____
Running:	_____	_____
Other:	_____	_____

WEIGHTLIFTING

4. Record your weightlifting goals.

	Weight (lb.)	Reps	Sets
Lat Pulldown	_____	_____	_____
Triceps	_____	_____	_____
Biceps	_____	_____	_____
Chest Press	_____	_____	_____
Shoulder Press	_____	_____	_____
Abdominals	_____	_____	_____
Quadriceps	_____	_____	_____
Hamstrings	_____	_____	_____
Calves	_____	_____	_____

FUTURE EXERCISE GOALS

5. What are your exercise goals for six months and a year from now?

Six months: _____

_____

Twelve months: _____

_____

Chapter 8

Keeping the Promise

Your resolution will always be important! Your promises will never keep themselves. There will never be a magic pill that jumps out of your body and closes the refrigerator door. You will always need to exert some resolve to achieve and maintain a healthy body weight. Remember, the Resolution Diet isn't about "going on" a diet. It's about developing a plan of nutrition and exercise for a lifetime.

So how will you maintain your weight loss over the long term? Willpower itself is never enough in the long run. The power of your mind, using well-thought-out new resolutions to constantly improve yourself, is the key to success.

In this chapter, I am going to give you strategies that will help you maintain your healthy habits, even in the face of an unhealthy food environment. You will learn skills that will help you remain resolute in different situations, so that you do not abandon your plan. These skills include not becoming overconfident, tailoring your individual approach, and not letting your moods get in the way. They will help you be successful over the long haul. The profile in the back will help you concentrate on the areas that most concern you.

DON'T GET OVERCONFIDENT: PREVENTING RELAPSES

It is tempting, as you look in the mirror at the "new" you, to forget the "old" you. You feel that you are cured of the problem of excess body fat, and that you will never go back to the old you again. That's when temptation strikes. "Eat that pizza? Why not? I've lost my weight, and I will probably never gain it back." Wrong! This is exactly the type of thinking that has caused hundreds of my patients to regain lost weight. By forgetting where you came from, you lose your resolution. In order to keep your promise, you must always remember that you have the potential to regain *all* the weight you have lost.

Scientists have developed a theory, drawn from studies of smoking and alcohol cessation, called relapse prevention. This theory emphasizes becoming conscious of your unhealthy behaviors when they happen, so that you can plan to avoid them in the future.

Whenever you make a mistake, it is called a lapse. This will happen at one time or another to all of us, including me. (I am amused at how people stare at my plate to see what I am eating, or attempt to get me to eat birthday cakes or sweet desserts.) Expect to make some mistakes. But while no one is perfect, you should realize these *are* mistakes.

A repeated lapse is called a relapse. Now you knew better, and did it anyway. However, if you are aware of each lapse and try to figure out what caused it, then you can prevent a relapse. Is stress creeping into your life? Are you staying too long in the kitchen after dinner? Finding out what's behind the lapses is critical, since a series of relapses combine to form a collapse, in which you throw in the towel. To avoid getting anywhere near a total collapse, become aware of the lapses and practice relapse prevention.

AVOID YO-YO DIETING

Do you know people who complain about going on one failed diet after another? With each new diet, the plan starts out great but ends up not working. However, it's not the diets that aren't working. What actually happens is that the dieter finds a way to get around the new diet somehow, and the magic wears off. Old habits return unnoticed, and the weight follows. What's really amazing is that these dieters are ready to embrace the next fad diet as the final answer. A cycle of lapse-relapse-collapse occurs in these dieters. They never notice the lapse and relapse, though, so the collapse is unexpected.

To avoid this trap, be aware of your lapses. My patients often say they are aware of eating anything that they shouldn't be eating. I encourage this, because it tells me that they are conscious of their eating habits. Stay on top of your plan and you can avoid failing—the best defense is a good offense. By constantly setting new goals for yourself, you will always remain conscious of your eating habits.

DON'T EAT "NORMALLY": CONTROLLING YOUR IMPULSES

Many of my patients feel that they should be able to eat "normally" like everyone else. In fact, the rest of our society is not eating "normally" at all. There is nothing normal about the typical American diet. Some people have the genes to get away with eating a high-fat, high-sweet diet, but you are not one of them! The poor eating habits of these people will show up in other diseases, but you are fortunate in showing all the extra calories you eat. Since the fat you eat is the fat you wear, you will have to stick with the Resolution Diet for the rest of your life. Remember, it is not a deprivation diet, but a set of better choices that taste good.

Controlling your impulse to eat "normally" is one key to controlling binge eating and other self-destructive habits that cause you to regain weight. Stimulus control requires planning. For example, I was recently on an airplane when the stewardess started rolling a cart with hot fudge sundaes down the aisle. I realized that this was a high-risk situation, because I would want one when she offered it. I began to practice self-talk: "Say no, say no, say no . . . ." She arrived at my seat. I said, "No thank you." As she wheeled the cart away I felt a moment of regret, but then I mentally congratulated myself for being morally superior to those who gave in to the urge for a hot fudge sundae.

Some people would say that there is nothing wrong with indulging once in a while, but let's analyze that idea. There was no occasion being celebrated. I was on an airplane and they decided to present me with those unnecessary calories. If you have a dessert every time it shows up in the environment, pretty soon you will be adding enough calories to your diet to sabotage your resolution. Practice self-talk and you will practice the skill of refusing unnecessary fat and calories.

RELAX CONTROL WHERE YOU CAN

I am often asked, "Will I have to eat this way forever?" The answer is yes and no. Yes—you are never going back to regularly eating those trigger foods again. No—you can eat whatever you want once in a great while and it won't hurt you. The key is in determining what "once in a great while" means. Some people can have one or two glasses of wine with dinner and leave it at that. Others have to go on to drink the whole bottle. As they do, they lose control of their eating habits and finish up with a rich dessert. Some people can eat Chinese food or red meat once a year and have no problem, but others will inevitably go on eating these foods once or twice a week, a rate that can affect calorie intake.

You have to know yourself. If eating trigger foods changes your diet, don't rationalize this behavior. Resolve to change it! There are many resolutions you will need to make as you go through life, but you will always need to eat. As you think about the foods you eat, shape your diet and make new resolutions to keep the promise over the long term.

There will be some areas where you can relax control, giving you the energy you need to tackle other areas. For example, when you reach your target weight, you will no longer need to eat less than your maintenance level of calories (see the chart on page 30). This means you can gradually increase your calorie intake by 500 to 1,000 calories, depending on whether you were losing 1 or 2 pounds per week when you were sticking with your plan 100 percent of the time. There are also all gradations of change in between maintaining your weight and losing the amount you have been losing. It is OK to take a break from losing weight even before you have reached your target. Let's say there is a lot going on at work, or you have a sudden tragedy, or illness hits your family. Put your diet on hold, and eat a little more. Just don't go back to any of the trigger foods. Control your urges to eat, and especially resist the idea of feeling sorry for yourself and eating. You won't feel any better by going back to your old habits, you'll just gain weight. Eating more of the right foods is OK at stressful times such as these. You can change your resolution to fit your situation.

DON'T LET YOUR MOODS GET IN THE WAY

It's natural to be in a bad mood every once in a while. Women often have this problem in the ten days before the menstrual period begins. This premenstrual syndrome is caused in part by a female hormone, progesterone, which is a mild depressant. Other people get depressed in the winter, when it gets dark during the day. Many of my patients get depressed when they are overstressed. This can be the result of burnout after taking on too much responsibility. And of course, bad moods sometimes hit for no apparent reason whatsoever. No matter why you are feeling low, don't feel sorry for yourself and start overeating again. Regaining the weight you worked so hard to lose won't improve your mood.

LEARN TO CONTROL YOUR STRESS

Do you know anyone who leads a stress-free life? Neither do I.

But stress does not have to automatically trigger inappropriate eating. The idea is to keep your stress levels down to a manageable level. Remember that exercise and adequate sleep are wonderful stress reducers. So is learning to take time for yourself, to give yourself the time you need to relax and let go for a while. If you don't take care of your needs, you will reach a point where you can't take care of anything else! In addition, learning stress-reduction techniques, such as meditation, can help you cut your stress levels no matter what the cause.

OBTAIN AND MAINTAIN SOCIAL SUPPORT

The most important thing in life is the network of relationships we all create for ourselves. When those closest to you don't support what you are doing, it becomes tough to maintain any new lifestyle behavior. Therefore building a social-support network is a vital part of maintaining your resolution. Humans are social animals. Whenever you go through an emotional experience, you tend to bond with those around you. The support of a loved one can make all the difference in keeping your promise.

Whenever there is a husband, wife, or companion waiting for a patient in my office, I invite them in for the consultation. I call this my "two-for-one special." In some instances, this procedure brings out the fact that a spouse is sabotaging the lifestyle efforts of the person who is trying to lose weight. Most commonly, an insecure husband keeps his attractive wife safely overweight by bringing her desserts every night. In other cases, wives use food as a way to rebel against an overly controlling "executive" husband. In these cases, I encourage an open discussion of the planned lifestyle changes. Since the spouse or companion and the patient eat together, shop together, and cook together, they should support each other in this lifestyle change. That may mean doing the Resolution Diet together. Or it may involve just respecting a loved one's choice, and working as a supportive spouse to encourage the development of new habits and the dropping of old habits.

People who are alone have a tougher problem. Loneliness can be a tremendous stimulus to overeating. Building relationships begins with friendships. I have even seen friendships develop between patients who met in my waiting room and formed support teams. Some organizations, such as Overeaters Anonymous, have used this system to provide a "buddy" who calls by phone. Finding a weight-loss partner if you are not married or joining a support group such as Overeaters Anonymous can be a key strategy in keeping your promise.

The Internet provides a way to find support from anywhere, even if you are living somewhere where it would be difficult to find a supportive partner. The Resolution Diet website—resolutiondiet.com—is a place where you can find a supportive buddy on-line. This site has been established to provide you the opportunity to register yourself with us, and to find friends anywhere in the country who can give you support any time of the day or night.

REMEMBER THAT EXERCISE IS A LIFELONG LIFESTYLE

Time is on your side when it comes to exercise. This is a lifetime commitment, just like your eating plan. Don't expect results after the first workout, but you should start feeling better right away. You will have more energy, sleep better, and feel less stressed. Keeping your regular commitment to exercise is very important, because it is the only way to burn off body fat and keep it off. Be consistent. (You may, for various reasons, feel more comfortable exercising at home with a friend.) Every time you stop, deconditioning of the muscles begins to occur within several weeks, and what's worse, you will start to regain body fat. By maintaining your exercise habit, you will keep the weight off permanently.

MONITOR AND REWARD YOURSELF

Keep a record of how you are doing. Every few weeks after you reach your goal, you should weigh yourself and record the results in a little book or in a computer file. By keeping a record, you will be monitoring your progress. A weight regain of greater than 10 percent of your total weight, or of half the weight you have lost, should trigger a complete overhaul and a new beginning to your Resolution Diet.

Over the years, among the thousands of patients I have seen, people often return to see me after they have regained significant weight over their minimum weight, but before they have regained all of their lost weight. This tells me that they are conscious of their weight gain, and I take this as a good sign.

Positive activities put joy in life, just as overwork and overstress result in burnout and depression. They can also serve as rewards for a job well done. Find an activity you can enjoy, such as golf, gardening, tennis, reading, painting, pottery, or taking nature walks. Make this hobby something that you identify with. By reading about the activity and getting more involved in it, you will provide a natural support for the effort of maintaining your lifestyle, diet, and exercise. You have seen bumper stickers that say, "The worst day of golf beats the best day at the office." This attitude provides a positive quality of life by providing something for you personally. One of the personality types that has the hardest time in terms of long-term maintenance is the "caretaker" personality. This is the person who takes care of everyone else, and takes care of herself or himself with food. If this describes you, having a strong interest or hobby counteracts this personality type by providing an opportunity for you to give to yourself.

MAKE NEW RESOLUTIONS TO SHAPE YOUR INDIVIDUAL APPROACH

I recently saw one of my male patients who had lost 17 pounds using meal replacements and the Resolution Diet, avoiding trigger foods to the best of his ability. He had a new problem. He told me that he felt flabby for the first time. I explained to him that he didn't exercise enough while he was losing weight, and that he probably lost both muscle and fat as the result of losing weight too quickly. However, he could now set a new exercise plan, one that included weightlifting, to build his muscle. This was particularly important for him because he had early diabetes, and the muscles he built would help prevent his diabetes from getting out of control. It would also help lower his levels of blood fats (triglyceride and cholesterol). So what we have is one resolution completed—losing weight—and a new resolution born out of this experience—gaining muscle. This new resolution will require continuing to eat the right foods and avoiding trigger foods, but taking in enough calories to build muscle over a three- to six-month period. This will include joining a gym and getting specific advice on how to build muscle. As he works on his new resolution, he will automatically be maintaining his original resolution.

You should do the same thing. As you work at improving your diet, don't ever think that you have finished the process. There is no end to the refinements you can make in your plan. By analyzing what you are eating, the types of exercise you are doing, and your stresses, you can tailor your approach and concentrate on those habits that need to be changed. By continually working on different aspects of your diet, exercise, and lifestyle, you will prevent any backsliding. So keep working as if you still have a long way to go.

ADMIT THAT EVERY NEGATIVE HAS A POSITIVE

No matter how destructive a habit is, there is often a perceived benefit that is maintaining that behavior. It may be a real struggle for you to change your eating and exercise habits for good. If that's the case, it may help to admit that overeating and underactivity have had positive benefits in other parts of your life. What are those benefits? If it is stress reduction, then how else could you reduce stress? Is to keep you from having to face social situations, problems in relationships, or your fears about work or personal life? How can you address these issues?

Analyze why you are tempted to overeat. This will help you stay on track.

MAINTAIN FOCUS, MOTIVATION, COMMITMENT, AND FOLLOW-THROUGH

Maintain focus. I have spent a lot of time with you defining your personal needs. The idea was to allow you to focus on what is important to you. If you have not focused yourself properly, go back to the chapters on diet and exercise, and define your needs. Visualize your goals. This is the first step in achieving them.

Stay motivated. Many different things can motivate behavior change. Fear is a motivator, such as if your doctor tells you that your excess body fat is threatening your health. However, years of research have shown that positive motivators are better. How you look in the mirror everyday is a stronger motivator than fear of illness. Find your motivation in your new shape and your new sense of well-being. Motivation will help you keep your resolution.

Make a commitment. Book an appointment with yourself for exercise. Write out your shopping list. Review the personal profiles at the end of each chapter, so that you will know what you need to work on and keep working on.

Follow through for a lifetime. Lots of us start and stop new diets all the time. I have patients who have started with me on seven different occasions. They usually come back before regaining all their weight, and are as successful the next time by simply starting the same plan again.

Remember: focus, motivation, commitment, follow-through. These are the keys to the Resolution Diet.

THE BOTTOM LINE

The hidden purpose of the Resolution Diet is to increase your self-esteem. Whether you are successful in every part of your life but this one, or are one of those people for whom nothing seems to work out, succeeding in losing weight and maintaining your weight loss is something you should feel good about. If you goof up, so what! Don't feel guilty or dejected. Figure out why you stopped. Write down the reason. Then go back to the beginning and start again. By simply working through this process, you will make gains. Give yourself permission to take it slowly sometimes, but don't change your basic habits.

If you ever learned to golf or play a musical instrument, you know how difficult it was. It didn't happen the very first time. So be kind and gentle with yourself, and you will gain the benefits of the Resolution Diet for the rest of your life.

Your Keeping-the-Promise
PROFILE

Answer the following sixteen questions to determine how you can keep your weight-loss promise to yourself.

PRACTICING RELAPSE CONTROL

1. How often have you lapsed in the past week?

2. Why did you lapse?

3. How can you prevent a relapse?

AVOIDING YO-YO DIETING

4. Have you been a yo-yo dieter in the past?

☐ Yes   ☐ No

5. If so, how can you prepare now to restart your diet, if you stop losing weight temporarily?

CONTROLLING IMPULSES

6. Have you recently been tempted to binge?

☐ Yes   ☐ No

7. What was the situation?

8. How did you handle it?

RELAXING CONTROL

9. On what special occasions would you like to relax control (without eating trigger foods)?

10. Are you in a situation right now in which you need to relax control? What is it?

CONTROLLING MOODS AND STRESS ·

11. What is your general mood now?
☐ Happy   ☐ Satisfied   ☐ Content
☐ Angry   ☐ Depressed   ☐ Guilty

12. What could you do to improve your outlook, if anything?

MAINTAINING SOCIAL SUPPORT

13. Who provides your social support network?

☐ Spouse/partner   ☐ Friend/relative

☐ Gym buddy   ☐ Coworker

14. How can you make this support work better?

☐ Telephone contact

☐ E-mail regularly

☐ Other

ADAPTING YOUR RESOLUTIONS

15. What were your original resolutions?

Diet _____

Exercise _____

Stress reduction _____

16. Are there any new resolutions you now feel are appropriate?

Diet _____

Exercise _____

Stress reduction _____

Conclusion

Bring It All Together and Make It Happen

How would you feel if you could walk through the grocery store without being drawn to the many high-fat, high-sweet foods that you ate and loved as a child? What if you felt free of cheese puffs, potato chips, corn chips, cookies, cakes, chocolates, cheeses, mayonnaise, high-fat salad dressings? What if you conquered your desires for all of them without feeling deprived? You would feel yourself to be in control of the urges that the advertising industry throws at you. You would control your environment by choosing the healthy foods and avoiding the unhealthy foods. You would ultimately come to the point where *you* are in control—not those snack foods.

My main message is simple: You can lose weight now and maintain that loss for the rest of your life. As a doctor, I know that the material in this book will help you lose weight. As a person who was overweight himself, I know that reading about weight loss and doing something about it is not the same thing. By working the principles and strategies in this book into the way you live your life, you can take back control of the way you eat.

There are many benefits you can attain by achieving a healthy weight, from being able to zip up your pants to avoiding a heart attack. I know, from my work with so many different people, that you have it in you to do this. That's true whether this is the first time you are losing weight or this is the latest of many weight-loss attempts. You cannot succeed if you don't at least try. You can succeed by setting your goals correctly, by knowing who you are, and by following a program you can live with. In this book, I have given you all the information you need to make a permanent change in not only your eating habits, but in your approach to exercise and stress reduction, and in your awareness of the high-fat world in which we live.

The key to understanding the Resolution Diet is that you are not temporarily giving up what you really want by using willpower to resist your desires. Instead, you are deciding on what is best for you, based on an understanding of why you eat, what you eat now, and how you can educate your palate to change permanently. In fact, you will finally be taking control of what you eat and the environment around you.

There are three basic principles that support the Resolution Diet. First, you need to restrict your fat intake and control your portion sizes through the use of meal replacements and portion-controlled meals, while avoiding trigger foods. Second, you need to engage in both aerobic and heavy resistance exercise if you want to maintain your weight loss. Third, you can change your behavior by using behavior modification techniques developed for other lifestyle changes, such as smoking cessation and alcoholism treatment. These are not my theories as a diet guru. I have simply put together in an understandable fashion the various nutrition and behavior messages that work. Yogi Berra is credited with saying, "Ninety-five percent of baseball is 50 percent psychology." The same can be said of the Resolution Diet.

Under some circumstances, the Resolution Diet by itself may not be enough. If you are drastically overweight, as discussed in Chapter 2, your weight problem may pose an imminent risk to your health. If that's the case, you need to see a doctor who specializes in weight problems, a specialty called bariatrics. He or she will be happy to hear that you are trying to lose weight, and will be able to adjust any medications you take for weight-associated problems, or to find you any additional help you may need. The doctor may discuss other approaches to weight loss, such as prescription drugs or even obesity surgery, that can be used together with the approaches you have read about in this book.

This book has not been about moderation, but rather about making definite changes. Trying to cut down on favorite foods comes a distant second to eliminating them altogether. You now know that a lapse in your resolution can lead to a relapse, which can lead to a collapse. The next time you see a trigger food you know you should not eat, don't think that just this once won't hurt you. You will end up quitting on the whole idea. Up until now, you have been told all foods are permissible in small quantities. I'm telling you that you must make a clean break with your old way of eating.

You have learned to educate your palate by taking control of all aspects of your diet. This involves controlling gratuitous fat and calories while optimizing fruit, vegetable, and grain intake. This is a common-sense approach that doesn't involve artificially counting fat grams, carbs, protein exchanges, or other nutrition numbers. Instead, you now understand that as long as you eat controlled portions of the right foods, your body will figure things out for itself. You don't have to sweat the small stuff. However, our diets have been so filled with extra calories, fat, and sugar that you will need to adjust your diet so that your body can respond. Restaurant eating, which makes up 60 percent of all meals for many of us, is a particularly important place to take control of your diet.

You have also learned that only you can design your personal Resolution Diet. Every one of us has different needs and desires. It has often been said that there are no junk foods, just junk diets. Well, I have news for you. If you put enough junk foods together, you have a junk diet! Make changes in the foods that count, use exercise to burn off calories, become aware of why and what you eat, and you will have a healthy diet that can help you achieve and maintain a healthy body weight, once and for all. If you have enough motivation, this will be the time you will succeed at keeping your resolution—the Resolution Diet.

I know that I cannot be there personally to motivate you. The promise you make to yourself next is a promise you must work towards keeping. You are the key. You must be the one who resolves to change. There is no treatment program or counselor who can do this without your willingness to move forward. This book lays out the steps you need to succeed at losing those unwanted pounds. Now, it is your turn. Fill out and sign the pledge on the next page. Use the profiles to guide the process, review this book when you need to, and use our website for information and support at http:\\www.resolutiondiet.com. Lose weight on your terms. Make the Resolution Diet your own.

Taking the
PLEDGE

I, _____,
(PRINT YOUR NAME HERE)

have read this book and believe that now is the
time to take responsibility for the way I eat. I
will create a weight-loss program, based upon
the principles in this book, that fits my lifestyle
and needs. I will use the appropriate strategies
in this book to achieve the target weight I have
set over the period of time I have allotted.

I can lose the weight and keep it off. I now
know how. I am taking Dr. Heber's Resolution
Diet Pledge.

Date:_____

Target Weight:_____

Target Date:_____

Signature:_____

Appendix A

Suggested Reading List

American Heart Association. *Fitting in Fitness: Hundreds of Simple Ways to Put More Physical Activity Into Your Life.* New York: Time Books, Random House, 1997.

Brownell KD, Wadden TA. *The LEARN Program for Weight Control.* Dallas: American Health Publishing Company, 1998.

Covey SR. *First Things First.* New York: Fireside, 1994.

Covey SR. *Principle-Centered Leadership.* New York: Fireside, 1990.

Covey SR. *Seven Habits of Highly Effective People.* New York: Simon & Schuster, 1989.

Ginsberg B, Milken M. *A Taste for Living.* New York: Time Warner Books, 1998.

Heber D. *Natural Remedies for a Healthy Heart.* Garden City Park, NY: Avery Publishing Group, 1998.

Ornish D. *Everyday Cooking With Dr. Dean Ornish.* New York: HarperCollins, 1996.

Pritikin R. *The Pritikin Weight Loss Breakthrough.* New York: Penguin/Putnam, 1998.

Weil A. *Spontaneous Healing.* New York: Fawcett Columbine, 1995.

Appendix B

Determining Your Body Mass Index

Want to know your body mass index (BMI), but the chart on pages 28–29 doesn't list your height? No problem. You can easily determine your own BMI using the following formula:

$$\frac{\text{Weight (pounds)}}{\text{Height (inches)}^2} \times 705 = \text{BMI}$$

To use this formula, just follow these steps. Let's assume, for the sake of this example, that you are 5 feet, 4 inches tall, and weigh 121 pounds.

1. First, calculate your height in inches, and square it—in other words, multiply the number by itself. In our example, your height is 64 inches. So:

$$64 \times 64 = 4{,}096$$

2. Now, write down your weight in pounds. In our example, your weight is 121 pounds.

3. Divide the smaller number (in this case, 121) by the larger number (4,096), rounding off your answer to the nearest hundredth:

$$121 \div 4{,}096 = .03$$

4. Multiply your final number—.03—by 705.

$$.03 \times 705 = 21$$

In this example, your BMI is 21.

Appendix C

A Two-Week Meal Plan

The two-week meal plan in this appendix is based on the 1,200- and 1,500-calorie plans on pages 72 and 73 in Chapter 4. I have supplied a cafeteria-style plan that includes fourteen breakfasts, lunches, and dinners (plus the afternoon snacks listed in Chapter 4). And to get you going, I have also supplied a day-by-day meal plan for one week that includes breakfasts, lunches, dinners, *and* snacks. I encourage you to explore the healthy, low-fat foods recommended in this book so you can start putting together your own meal plans.

CAFETERIA-STYLE MEAL PLAN

This plan lists breakfasts, lunches, and dinners for two weeks. Feel free to use all of the items listed, or to repeat a particular favorite several times a week. All shakes referred to are meal replacements. The dinners call for either 3 or 6 ounces of poultry or fish, depending on whether you are following the 1,200- or 1,500-calorie meal plan.

Breakfast Choices

1 chocolate shake mixed with 1 teaspoon instant coffee
1 medium orange

1 vanilla shake blended with 1 medium banana and a sprinkle
of nutmeg

1 vanilla shake blended with 1 cup strawberries (try using
frozen fruit—the shake will be extra thick and creamy)

1 vanilla shake blended with 1 medium peach and a dash of
nutmeg

1 vanilla shake blended with 1 medium banana and $^1/_4$ teaspoon orange extract

1 vanilla shake mixed with 1 teaspoon instant coffee and a few
drops almond extract
$^1/_2$ grapefruit

1 pineapple-orange shake blended with 1 medium banana

1 vanilla shake mixed with $^1/_2$ teaspoon peppermint extract
1 cup cubed melon

1 strawberry shake blended with 1 medium banana

1 vanilla shake mixed with $^1/_2$ teaspoon rum extract and a
sprinkle of nutmeg
$^1/_2$ grapefruit

3 herb-seasoned egg whites (scrambled in skillet sprayed with
cooking spray)
1 slice whole grain toast
1 cup cubed cantaloupe

1 cup high-fiber cold cereal
1 cup berries (your choice)
1 cup nonfat milk

1 cup cooked oatmeal, made with nonfat milk; sprinkle with cinnamon

1 medium orange

Lowfat French Toast: Beat together 3 egg whites. Dip 1 slice whole grain bread in egg whites; brown on both sides in skillet sprayed with cooking spray. Top with 1 sliced medium banana and a sprinkle of cinnamon

Lunch Choices

1 vanilla shake blended with 1 medium peach

1 small tomato and $1/2$ cup julienned bell pepper. Toss with balsamic vinegar, mustard, basil, salt, and pepper to taste

1 chocolate shake blended with 1 medium banana

$1/2$ cup each steamed broccoli and carrots, seasoned with garlic, ginger, and a splash of soy sauce

1 chocolate shake blended with 1 cup frozen whole strawberries

2 cups salad greens with seasoned rice vinegar

1 strawberry shake blended with 1 cup raspberries

2 cups salad greens with balsamic vinegar

1 pineapple-orange shake

2 cups salad greens with seasoned vinegar

1 cup cubed watermelon

1 chocolate shake blended with $1/2$ teaspoon almond extract

2 cups mixed salad greens with seasoned rice vinegar

1 medium banana

1 frozen vanilla shake topped with 1 cup fresh blueberries

2 cups salad greens with white wine vinegar and tarragon

1 vanilla shake mixed with few drops cherry and almond extracts

2 cups mixed salad greens with lemon and herbs

1 medium pear

1 frozen chocolate shake

2 cups mixed greens with seasoned vinegar

1 apple, baked with cinnamon

1 frozen meal replacement (your choice) topped with 1 cup mixed berries

Salad made with 1 cup romaine lettuce and 1 medium tomato dressed with seasoned rice vinegar

Grilled Chicken Sandwich: On 2 slices whole grain bread place 3 ounces grilled chicken breast and 2 cups salad greens seasoned with lemon and garlic

1 medium plum

Sandwich and Salad Combo: On 2 slices whole grain bread place 3 ounces roasted turkey breast, mustard, sliced tomato, and sliced cucumber

2 cups mixed greens with seasoned vinegar

1 medium pear

Grilled Seafood Salad: Top 2 cups mixed greens with 3 ounces grilled fish. Season with oil-free vinaigrette dressing

2 slices whole grain toast

$^1/_2$ grapefruit (try tossing the grapefruit sections into the salad)

Pita Pocket Sandwich: Stuff 1 whole grain pita bread with 3 ounces flaked tuna and 2 cups mixed greens. Add salsa, sprouts, and shredded carrots to taste

1 cup cubed melon

Dinner Choices

Grilled Fish Dinner: Grill 3 to 6 ounces firm fish, along with 2 cups red peppers and asparagus

1 7-ounce potato; bake or boil ahead of time, cut into 1-inch slices, and grill

2 cups tossed salad greens with lemon and dill

1 cup melon balls

Taco Salad: Make the salad with $1/2$ cup each cooked brown rice and black beans, plus 3 to 6 ounces cooked ground turkey breast seasoned with garlic, chili powder, oregano, and cumin on top of 2 cups salad greens. Top with salsa
2 cups steamed broccoli and carrots
1 frozen medium banana; peel, place on foil, and freeze

Chicken or Seafood Bowl: Top 1 cup steamed brown rice with 3 to 6 ounces chicken or fish grilled with teriyaki, plus 2 cups steamed broccoli, asparagus, peppers, carrots, and spinach
2 cups tossed salad greens with rice vinegar, ginger, and soy sauce
1 medium pear

Barbecue Dinner: Grill 3 to 6 ounces chicken breast with barbecue sauce
1 cup fresh yellow corn
2 cups steamed broccoli, spinach, and carrots with lemon
2 cups tossed salad greens with white wine vinegar
1 cup cubed watermelon

Baked Crunchy Fish: Coat 3 to 6 ounces sole or other white fish with crushed bran flakes and seafood seasoning, and bake
1 cup steamed spinach with roasted garlic
2 cups tossed salad greens with lemon
1 cup brown rice
1 medium apple, baked with cinnamon and cloves

Chopped Grilled Citrus Shrimp Salad: Place 3 to 6 ounces shrimp (marinated in citrus juices and grilled) atop 2 cups salad greens, $1/2$ cup each black beans and corn, and 2 cups chopped carrots, tomatoes, and peppers. Season with rice vinegar
1 poached pear with cinnamon

Pasta with Meatballs: Make meatballs with 3 to 6 ounces ground turkey breast, seasoned with oregano, salt, and pepper to taste. Broil, then mix with 1 cup heated stewed tomatoes. Place atop 1 cup cooked whole wheat pasta, add 1 cup steamed zucchini with basil
2 cups tossed salad greens with balsamic vinegar
1 cup fresh strawberries

Pasta Salad: Mix 1 cup cooked whole grain pasta with 3 to 6 ounces grilled shrimp and 2 cups steamed broccoli, bell pepper, and carrots. Season with fat-free vinaigrette
2 cups tossed salad greens with balsamic vinegar
1 medium orange

Chicken Fajitas: Grill 3 to 6 ounces chicken breast strips seasoned with taco seasoning. Mix with $1^1/_2$ cups grilled bell pepper and onion strips, $^1/_2$ cup salsa, and shredded lettuce. Divide among 3 corn tortillas
2 cups tossed salad greens with balsamic vinegar
1 cup strawberries

Quick Minestrone Soup: In water or broth, heat together 3 to 6 ounces cooked chicken breast, 1 cup cooked pasta, 1 cup each tomato and zucchini. Season with oregano, salt, and pepper to taste
2 cups tossed salad greens with balsamic vinegar
1 cup berries (your choice)

Roasted Turkey Dinner: Roast 3 to 6 ounces fresh turkey breast along with 1 medium potato that is sliced, sprayed with cooking spray, and sprinkled with salt and pepper
2 cups steamed broccoli and cauliflower, seasoned with lemon and garlic
2 cups tossed salad greens with seasoned vinegar
1 medium banana

Turkey Burger: Broil a burger made with 3 to 6 ounces of ground turkey. Place on 1 whole wheat hamburger bun with sliced lettuce, tomato, and onion

2 cups tossed salad greens with seasoned vinegar

1 cup cubed cantaloupe

Sole and Spinach: Bake 3 to 6 ounces fresh sole, seasoned with lemon, salt, and pepper, and place on a bed of 1 cup cooked spinach

2 cups tossed salad greens with 1 small tomato and $1/2$ cup bell pepper and seasoned vinegar

1 cup brown rice

1 medium plum

Fish Kabobs: On skewers, string 3 to 6 ounces firm fish with 2 cups vegetables (peppers, zucchini, tomato). Season with teriyaki and grill

1 7-ounce baked potato

2 cups tossed salad greens with seasoned vinegar

1 cup mixed berries

DAY-BY-DAY MEAL PLAN

This plan provides a complete guide to meals for one week, including all breakfasts, lunches, snacks, and dinners. All shakes referred to are meal replacements. For each snack, the first choice is part of the 1,200-calorie meal plan, while the second choice is part of the 1,500-calorie plan (which includes your choice of shake). The dinners call for either 3 or 6 ounces of poultry or fish, depending on whether you are following the 1,200- or 1,500-calorie plan.

Day One

Breakfast: 1 chocolate shake mixed with 1 teaspoon instant
             coffee
             1 medium orange

Lunch: **Grilled Chicken Sandwich:** On 2 slices whole grain
             bread place 3 ounces grilled chicken breast and 2
             cups salad greens seasoned with lemon and garlic
             1 medium plum

Snack: 1 banana plus 1 caramel popcorn rice cake
             1 banana plus 2 caramel popcorn rice cakes plus
             1 shake

Dinner: **Grilled Fish Dinner:** Grill 3 to 6 ounces firm fish,
             along with 2 cups red peppers and asparagus
             1 7-ounce potato; bake or boil ahead of time, cut into
             1-inch slices, and grill
             2 cups tossed salad greens with lemon and dill
             1 cup melon balls

  Day Two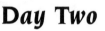

Breakfast: 1 cup high-fiber cold cereal
             1 cup berries (your choice)
             1 cup nonfat milk

Lunch: 1 vanilla shake blended with 1 medium peach
             1 small tomato and $\frac{1}{2}$ cup julienned bell pepper.
             Toss with balsamic vinegar, mustard, basil, salt,
             and pepper to taste

Snack: 1 cup mixed berries plus 1 apple cinnamon rice cake
             1 cup mixed berries plus 2 apple cinnamon rice
             cakes plus 1 shake

Dinner: **Taco Salad:** Make the salad with $1/2$ cup each cooked brown rice and black beans, plus 3 to 6 ounces cooked ground turkey breast seasoned with garlic, chili powder, oregano, and cumin on top of 2 cups salad greens. Top with salsa

2 cups steamed broccoli and carrots

1 frozen medium banana; peel, place on foil, and freeze

  Day Three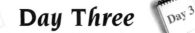

Breakfast: 1 vanilla shake blended with 1 medium banana and a sprinkle of nutmeg

Lunch: **Sandwich and Salad Combo:** On 2 slices whole grain bread place 3 ounces roasted turkey breast, mustard, sliced tomato, and sliced cucumber

2 cups mixed greens with seasoned vinegar

1 medium pear

Snack: 1 cup cubed watermelon/cantaloupe plus 1 popcorn rice cake

1 cup cubed melon plus 2 popcorn rice cakes plus 1 shake

Dinner: **Chicken or Seafood Bowl:** Top 1 cup steamed brown rice with 3 to 6 ounces chicken or fish grilled with teriyaki, plus 2 cups steamed broccoli, asparagus, peppers, carrots, and spinach

2 cups tossed salad greens with rice vinegar, ginger, and soy sauce

1 medium pear

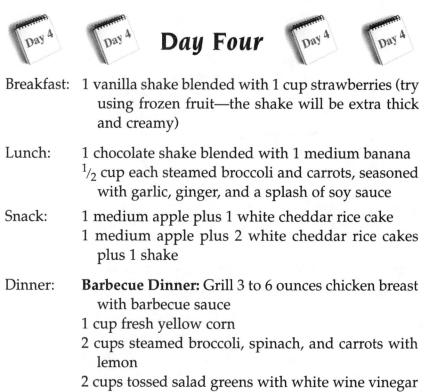

Day Four

Breakfast: 1 vanilla shake blended with 1 cup strawberries (try using frozen fruit—the shake will be extra thick and creamy)

Lunch: 1 chocolate shake blended with 1 medium banana
$1/2$ cup each steamed broccoli and carrots, seasoned with garlic, ginger, and a splash of soy sauce

Snack: 1 medium apple plus 1 white cheddar rice cake
1 medium apple plus 2 white cheddar rice cakes plus 1 shake

Dinner: **Barbecue Dinner:** Grill 3 to 6 ounces chicken breast with barbecue sauce
1 cup fresh yellow corn
2 cups steamed broccoli, spinach, and carrots with lemon
2 cups tossed salad greens with white wine vinegar
1 cup cubed watermelon

  ## Day Five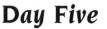

Breakfast: 1 vanilla shake blended with 1 medium peach and a dash of nutmeg

Lunch: 1 chocolate shake blended with 1 cup frozen whole strawberries
2 cups salad greens with seasoned rice vinegar

Snack: 1 medium orange plus 1 nacho cheese rice cake
1 medium orange plus 2 nacho cheese rice cakes plus 1 shake

Dinner: **Baked Crunchy Fish:** Coat 3 to 6 ounces sole or other white fish with crushed bran flakes and seafood seasoning, and bake
1 cup steamed spinach with roasted garlic
2 cups tossed salad greens with lemon
1 cup brown rice
1 medium apple, baked with cinnamon and cloves

  Day Six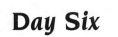

Breakfast: **Lowfat French Toast:** Beat together 3 egg whites. Dip 1 slice whole grain bread in egg whites; brown on both sides in skillet sprayed with cooking spray. Top with 1 sliced medium banana and a sprinkle of cinnamon

Lunch: 1 strawberry shake blended with 1 cup raspberries
2 cups salad greens with balsamic vinegar

Snack: 1 medium plum plus 1 white cheddar rice cake
1 medium plum plus 2 white cheddar rice cakes plus 1 shake

Dinner: **Chopped Grilled Citrus Shrimp Salad:** Place 3 to 6 ounces shrimp (marinated in citrus juices and grilled) atop 2 cups salad greens, $1/2$ cup each black beans and corn, and 2 cups chopped carrots, tomatoes, and peppers. Season with rice vinegar
1 poached pear with cinnamon

Day Seven

Breakfast: 1 vanilla shake blended with 1 medium banana and
            $^1/_4$ teaspoon orange extract

Lunch: 1 pineapple-orange shake
            2 cups salad greens with seasoned vinegar
            1 cup cubed watermelon

Snack: 1 medium peach plus 1 rice cake
            1 medium peach plus 2 rice cakes plus 1 shake

Dinner: **Pasta with Meatballs:** Make meatballs with 3 to
            6 ounces ground turkey breast, seasoned with
            oregano, salt, and pepper to taste. Broil, then
            mix with 1 cup heated stewed tomatoes. Place
            atop 1 cup cooked whole wheat pasta, add 1 cup
            steamed zucchini with basil
            2 cups tossed salad greens with balsamic vinegar
            1 cup fresh strawberries

References

Preface

Becker MH. The health belief model and personal health behavior. *Health Education Monograph* 2:324–473, 1974.

Friedman MA, Brownell KD. Psychological correlates of obesity: moving to the next research generation. *Psychological Bulletin* 117:3–20, 1995.

Gortmaker SI, Must A, Perrin JM, Sobol AM, Dietz WH. Social and economic consequences of overweight in adolescence and young adulthood. *New England Journal of Medicine* 329:1008–1012, 1993.

Kuczmarski RJ, Flegal KM, Campbell SM, Johnson CL. Increasing prevalence of overweight among US adults. *Journal of the American Medical Association* 272:205–211, 1994.

Neel JV. Thrifty genotype: the hunter-gatherer's friend. *American Journal of Human Genetics* 14:353–362, 1962.

Wadden TA, Wingate BJ. Compassionate treatment of the obese individual. In Brownell KD, Fairburn CG (eds). *Comprehensive Textbook of Eating Disorders and Obesity*. New York: Guilford Press, 1995, pp. 564–571.

Introduction

Heber D, Ashley JM, McCarthy WJ, Chang CJ, Elashoff R. Assessment of adherence to a low-fat diet for breast cancer prevention. *Preventive Medicine* 21:218–227, 1992.

Heber D, Ashley JM, Wang HJ, Elashoff RM. Clinical evaluation of a minimal intervention meal replacement regimen for weight reduction. *Journal of the American College of Nutrition* 6:608–614, 1994.

Institute of Medicine. *Weighing the Options: Criteria for Evaluating Weight Management Programs.* Washington, DC: U.S. Government Printing Office, 1995.

NIH Technology Assessment Panel. Methods of voluntary weight loss and control. *Annals of Internal Medicine* 199:764–770, 1993.

Yetiv JZ. *Popular Nutritional Practices: A Scientific Appraisal.* Toledo, OH: Popular Medicine Press, 1986, pp. 274–285.

Chapter 1

A Step-By-Step Weight-Loss Resolution

Blackburn GL, Kanders BS. *Obesity: Pathophysiology, Psychology and Treatment.* New York: Chapman and Hall, 1994.

Blair SN. Evidence for success of exercise in weight loss and control. *Annals of Internal Medicine* 119:702–706, 1993.

Foreyt JP, Goodrick KG. Evidence for success of behavior modification in weight loss and control. *Annals of Internal Medicine* 119:698–701, 1993.

National Institutes of Health; National Heart, Lung and Blood Institute. Clinical guidelines on the identification, evaluation and treatment of overweight and obesity in adults, 1998.

Ni Murchu C, Margetts BM, Speller VM. Applying the stages-of-change model to dietary change. *Nutrition Reviews* 55:10–16, 1997.

Weinseir RL, Wadden TA, Ritenbaugh C, et al. Recommended therapeutic guidelines for professional weight control programs. *American Journal of Clinical Nutrition* 40:865–872, 1984.

Chapter 2

Getting Ready to Lose Weight

Campfield LA, Smith FJ, Guisez Y, Devos R, Burn P. Recombinant mouse ob protein: evidence for a peripheral signal linking adiposity and central neural networks. *Science* 269:546–549, 1995.

Cloninger CR, Rice J, Reich T. Multifactorial inheritance with cultural transmission and associative mating II. A general model of combined polygenic and cultural inheritance. *American Journal of Human Genetics* 31:176–198, 1979.

Cooper PJ, Fairburn CG. The depressive symptoms of bulimia nervosa. *British Journal of Psychiatry* 148:268–274, 1986.

Dattilo AM, Kris-Etherton PM. Effects of weight reduction on blood lipids and lipoproteins: a meta-analysis. *American Journal of Clinical Nutrition* 56:320–328, 1992.

Dustan HP. Hypertension in obese patients. *Annals of Internal Medicine* 103:1047–1049, 1985.

Dye L, Blundell JA. Menstrual cycle and appetite control: implications for weight reduction. *Human Reproduction* 12:1142–1151, 1997.

Frank A. Futility and avoidance: medical professionals in the treatment of obesity. *Journal of the American Medical Association* 269:2132–2133, 1993.

Geiselman PJ. Sugar-induced hyperphagia: is hyperinsulinemia, hypoglycemia, or any other factor a "necessary" condition ? *Appetite* 11(Suppl 1):26–34, 1988.

Gibbs, WW. Gaining on fat. *Scientific American* pp. 88–94, August 1996.

Goldstein D. Beneficial health effects of modest weight loss. *International Journal of Obesity* 16: 397–415, 1992.

Halaas JL, Gajiwala KS, Maffei M, Barone M, Leopold L, Friedman JM. Weight reducing effects of the plasma protein encoded by the obese gene. *Science* 269:540–543, 1995.

Hamer DH, Copeland P. *Living With Our Genes: Why They Matter More Than You Think.* New York: Doubleday, 1998.

Hartz AJ, Rupley CC, Rimm AA. The association of girth measurements with disease in 73,532 women. *Public Health Reports* 119:71–80, 1975.

Heber D, Ingles S, Ashley JM, Maxwell MH, Lyons RF, Elashoff RM. Clinical detection of sarcopenic obesity by bioelectrical impedance analysis. *American Journal of Clinical Nutrition* 64:472S–477S, 1996.

Hubert HB, Feinleib M, McNamara PM, et al. Obesity as an independent risk factor for cardiovascular disease: a 26-year follow-up of participants in the Framingham heart study. *Circulation* 67:968–977, 1983.

Marcus BH, Rakowski W, Rossi JS. Assessing motivational readiness and decision making for exercise. *Health Psychology* 11:257–261, 1992.

Mifflin, Mark D, St Jeor S, Hill LA, Scott BJ, Daugherty SA, Koh YO. A new predictive equation for resting energy expenditure in healthy individuals. *American Journal of Clinical Nutrition* 51:241–247, 1990.

O'Brien SN, Welter BH, Mantzke KA, Price TM. Identification of progesterone receptor in human subcutaneous adipose tissue. *Journal of Clinical Endocrinology and Metabolism* 83:509–513, 1998.

Quesenberry CP, Caan B, Jacobson A. Obesity, health services use, and health care costs among members of a health maintenance organization. *Archives of Internal Medicine* 158:466–472, 1998.

Rebuffe-Scrive M, Eldh J, Halfstrom LO, et al. Metabolism of mammary, abdominal, and femoral adipocytes in women before and after menopause. *Metabolism* 35:793–797, 1986.

Rodin J, Silberstein L, Streigel-Moore R. Women and weight: a normative discontent. In Sonderegger TB (ed). *Nebraska Symposium on Motivation: Psychology and Gender.* Lincoln: University of Nebraska Press, 1984, pp. 267–307.

Rohner-Jeanrenaud E, Jeanrenaud B. Central nervous system and body weight regulation. *Annals of Endocrinology* (Paris) 58:137–142, 1997.

Stunkard AJ, Sorenson TIA, Harris C. Adoption study of human obesity. *New England Journal of Medicine* 314:193–198, 1986.

Vague J. Degree of masculine differentiation of obesities. Factor determining predisposition to diabetes, atherosclerosis, gout, and uric calculous disease. *American Journal of Clinical Nutrition* 4:20–34, 1956.

Warren MP, Van de Wiele RL. Clinical and metabolic features of anorexia nervosa. *American Journal of Obstetrics and Gynecology* 117:435–441, 1973.

Wing RR, Koeske R, Epstein LH, et al. Long-term effects of modest weight loss in type II diabetic patients. *Archives of Internal Medicine* 147:1749–1753, 1987.

Wing RR, Matthews KA, Kuller LH, et al. Weight gain at the time of menopause. *Archives of Internal Medicine* 151:97–102, 1991.

Zhang Y, Proenca R, Maffei M, Barone M, Leopold L, Friedman JM. Positional cloning of the mouse obese gene and its human homologue. *Nature* 372:425–432, 1994.

Chapter 3
The Trigger Food Strategy

Block G, Clifford C, Naughton M, Henderson M, McAdams M. A brief dietary screen for high fat intake. *Journal of Nutritional Education* 21:199–207, 1989.

Brownell KD, Rodin J. Medical metabolic and psychological effects of weight cycling. *Archives of Internal Medicine* 154:1325–1330, 1994.

Campbell MK, DeVellis BM, Strecher VJ, Ammerman AS, DeVellis RF, Sandler RS. The impact of message tailoring on dietary behavior change for disease prevention in primary care settings. *American Journal of Public Health* 84:783–787, 1993.

Marcus MD, Wing RR, Lamparski DM. Binge eating and dietary restraint in obese patients. *Addictive Behaviors* 10:163–168, 1985.

Mattes RD. Fat preference and adherence to a reduced-fat diet. *American Journal of Clinical Nutrition* 57:373–381, 1993.

Rolls BJ. Carbohydrates, fats and satiety. *American Journal of Clinical Nutrition* 61:960S–967S, 1995.

Chapter 4
Meal Replacements and Portion-Controlled Foods

Ditschuneit HH, Flechtner-Mors M, Adler G. Metabolic and weight loss effects of long-term dietary intervention in obese subjects. *American Journal of Clinical Nutrition,* 1999 (at press).

Ditschuneit HH, Flechtner-Mors M, Adler G. The effectiveness of meal replacement with diet shakes on long-term weight loss and weight maintenance (abstract). Eighth International Congress on Obesity, Paris, 1998.

Flatt JP. Use and storage of carbohydrate and fat. *American Journal of Clinical Nutrition* 61:952S–959S, 1995.

Heber D, Ashley JM, Wang HJ, Elashoff RM. Clinical evaluation of a minimal intervention meal replacement regimen for weight reduction. *Journal of the American College of Nutrition* 6:608–614, 1994.

Lichtman SW, Pisarska K, Berman ER, Pestone M, Dowling H, Offenbacher E, Weisel H, Heshka S, Matthews DE, Heymsfield SB. Discrepancy between self-reported and actual caloric intake and exercise in obese subjects. *New England Journal of Medicine* 327:1893–1898, 1992.

Lissner L, Levitsky DA, Strupp BJ, Kalkwarf HJ, Roe DA. Dietary fat and the regulation of energy intake in human subjects. *American Journal of Clinical Nutrition* 46:886–892, 1987.

Rothacker D. Five-year weight control with meal replacements comparison with background in rural Wisconsin (abstract). Eighth International Congress on Obesity, Paris, 1998.

Shah M, McGovern P, French S, Baxter J. Comparison of a low-fat ad libitium complex carbohydrate diet with a low energy diet in moderately obese women. *American Journal of Clinical Nutrition* 59:980–984, 1994.

Chapter 5
Educating Your Palate

Anderson JW, Johnstone BM, Cook-Newell ME. Meta-analysis of the effects of soy protein intake on serum lipids. *New England Journal of Medicine* 333:276–282, 1995.

Bagga D, Capone S, Wang HJ, Heber D, Lill M, Chap L, Glaspy JA. Dietary modulation of omega 3/omega 6 polyunsaturated fatty acid ratios in patients with breast cancer. *Journal of the National Cancer Institute* 89:1123–1131, 1997.

Delargy HJ, O'Sullivan KR, Fletcher RJ, Blundell JE. Effects of amount and type of dietary fibre (soluble and insoluble) on short-term control of appetite. *International Journal of Food Science and Nutrition* 48:67–77, 1997.

Dickinson A. Optimal Nutrition for Good Health: The Benefits of Nutrition Supplements. Council for Responsible Nutrition, Washington, DC, 1998.

Dietary Guidelines Advisory Committee. *Report of the Dietary Guidelines Advisory Committee on the Dietary Guidelines for Americans.* U.S. Department of Agriculture, Human Nutrition Information Services, 1990.

Eaton SB, Konner M. Paleolithic nutrition: a consideration of its nature and current implications. *New England Journal of Medicine* 312:283–289, 1985.

Gorbach SL, Morrill-LaBrode A, Woods MN, Dwyer JT, Selles WD, Henderson M, Insull W, Goldman S, Thompson D, Clifford C, Sheppard L. Changes in food patterns during a low-fat dietary intervention in women. *Journal of the American Dietetic Association* 90:802–809, 1990.

Hathcock J. Vitamins and minerals: efficacy and safety. *American Journal of Clinical Nutrition* 66:427–437, 1997.

Jenkins D. Wholemeal versus wholegrain breads: proportion of whole wheat or cracked grain and glycemic index. *British Medical Journal* 297:958, 1988.

National Academy of Sciences, National Research Council, Food and Nutrition Board. *Diet and Health Implications for Reducing Chronic Disease Risk.* Washington, DC: National Academy Press, 1989.

Sims LS. *The Politics of Fat.* New York: M.E. Sharpe, 1998.

Suzuki M. Simultaneous ingestion of fat and sucrose may contribute to development of obesity: a larger body fat accumulation as compared with their separate ingestion. *Federation Proceedings* 45:481, 1986.

Ursin G, Ziegler RG, Subar AF, Graubard BI, Haile RW, Hoover R. Dietary patterns associated with a low-fat diet in the National Health Examination Follow-Up Study. Identification of potential confounders for epidemiologic analyses. *American Journal of Epidemiology* 137:916–927, 1993.

U.S. Department of Health and Human Services, Public Health Service. *The Surgeon General's Report on Diet and Health.* Washington, DC: U.S. Government Printing Office, 1988.

Chapter 6
Living the Resolution Diet

Fishbein M, Ajzen I. *Belief, Attitude, Intention, and Behavior: An Introduction to Theory and Research.* Reading MA: Addison Wesley, 1975.

Klem ML, Wing RR, McGuire MT, Seagle HM, Hill JO. A descriptive study of individuals successful at long-term maintenance of substantial weight loss. *American Journal of Clinical Nutrition* 66:239–246, 1997.

Sallis JF, Hovell MF, Hofstetter CR, Elder JP, Hackley M, Caspersen CJ, Powell KE. Distance between homes and exercise related to frequency of exercise among San Diego residents. *Public Health Reports* 105:179–185, 1990.

Urban N, White E, Anderson GL, Curry S, Kristal AR. Correlates of maintenance of a low-fat diet among women in the Women's Health Trial. *Preventive Medicine* 21:279–291, 1992.

Chapter 7
Get the Exercise and Stress-Reduction Habits

American Heart Association. *Fitting in Fitness.* New York: Times Books, 1997.

Blair SN, Haskell WL, Ho P, et al. Assessment of habitual physical activity by a seven day recall in a community survey and controlled experiments. *American Journal of Epidimology* 122:794, 1985.

King NA, Blundell JA. High-fat foods overcome the energy expenditure induced by high-intensity cycling or running. *European Journal of Clinical Nutrition* 49:114–123, 1995.

McCardle WD, Katch FI, Katch VL. *Essentials of Exercise Physiology.* Philadelphia: Lea and Febiger, 1994.

Mitchell SL, Epstein LH. Changes in taste and satiety in dietary-restrained women following stress. *Physiology and Behavior* 60:495–499, 1996.

Ossip-Klein DJ, Doyne EJ, Bowman ED, Osborn KM, McDougall-Wilson IB, Neimeyer RA. Effects of running or weightlifting on self-concept in clinically depressed women. *Journal of Consulting and Clinical Psychology* 57:158–161, 1997.

Yeung RR. The acute effects of exercise on mood state. *Journal of Psychosomatic Research* 40:123–141, 1996.

Chapter 8
Keeping the Promise

Brownell KD, Wadden TA. *The LEARN Program for Weight Control.* Dallas: American Health Publishing Company, 1998.

Lorenz RA, Bubb J, Davis D, Jacobson A, Jannasch K, Kramer J, Lipps J, Schlundt D. Changing behavior: practical lessons from the Diabetes Control and Complications Trial. *Diabetes Care* 19:648–652, 1996.

Marlatt GA, Gordon JR. Determinants of relapse: implications for maintenance of behavior change. In Davidson P, Davidson S. (eds.) *Behavioral Medicine: Changing Lifestyles.* New York: Bruner/Mazel, 1980, pp. 410–452.

Prochaska, JO, DiClemente CC. Stages and processes of self-change for smoking: toward an integrative model of change. *Journal of Consulting and Clinical Psychology* 51:390–395, 1992.

Strecher, VJ, Becker MH, Kirscht J, Eraker SA, Graham-Tomasi RP. Psychological aspects of changes in cigarette smoking behavior. *Patient Education and Counseling* 7:249–262, 1985.

Index